MCQs for the Paediat

Matthew Lulyag

01233 722000

vauxhall
R. 809 XKE

22:30

C 896 CKN

Toyota

Engine 1.8 00
size

07786 93331
01303 246473

N² 077 900 86267

For David

For Churchill Livingstone

Commissioning Editor: Timothy Horne
Project Editor: Janice Urquhart
Copy Editor: Isla MacLean
Project Controller: Kay Hunston
Design Direction: Erik Bigland

MCQs for the Paediatric MRCP Part 1

A. P. Winrow
BSc(Hons) MB BS MRCP(UK)
Consultant Paediatrician, Kingston Hospital, Surrey, UK

G. Supramaniam
MSc MB BS FRCP
Consultant Paediatrician, Watford General Hospital, Hertfordshire, UK

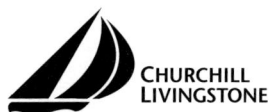

NEW YORK EDINBURGH LONDON MADRID MELBOURNE
SAN FRANCISCO TOKYO 1996

CHURCHILL LIVINGSTONE
Medical Division of Pearson Professional Limited

Distributed in the United States of America by
Churchill Livingstone Inc., 650 Avenue of the Americas,
New York, N.Y. 10011, and by associated companies,
branches and representatives throughout the world.

© Pearson Professional Limited 1996

All rights reserved. No part of this publication may
be reproduced, stored in a retrieval system, or
transmitted in any form or by any means,
electronic, mechanical, photocopying, recording or
otherwise, without either the prior permission of the
publishers (Churchill Livingstone, Robert Stevenson
House, 1–3 Baxter's Place, Leith Walk, Edinburgh
EH1 3AF), or a licence permitting restricted copying
in the United Kingdom issued by the Copyright
Licensing Agency Ltd, 90 Tottenham Court Road,
London W1P 9HE.

First published 1996

ISBN 0 443 05354 5

British Library Cataloguing in Publication Data
A catalogue record for this book is available from the British Library

Library of Congress Cataloging in Publication Data
A catalog record for this book is available from the Library of Congress

Medical knowledge is constantly changing. As new information becomes available, changes in treatment, procedures, equipment and the use of drugs become necessary. The authors and the publishers have, as far as it is possible, taken care to ensure that the information given in the text is accurate and up to date. However, readers are strongly advised to confirm that the information, especially with regard to drug usage, complies with current legislation and standards of practice.

The
publisher's
policy is to use
**paper manufactured
from sustainable forests**

Printed in Hong Kong
NPC/01

Contents

Preface	vii
1. Endocrinology	1
2. Infections	11
3. Neonatology	23
4. Development	37
5. Immunizations	39
6. Molecular biology	43
7. Immunology	47
8. Dermatology	51
9. Child abuse	55
10. Haematology and oncology	59
11. Metabolism	69
12. Neurology	77
13. Psychosocial paediatrics	89
14. Children's Act	91
15. Rheumatology and orthopaedics	93
16. Statistics	101
17. Pharmacology	103
18. Respirology	111
19. Embryology	129
20. Nephrology	137
21. Liver and gastroenterology	147
22. Diabetes	163
23. Genetics	169
24. Cardiology	175
Index	183

Preface

No longer is the paediatrician in training expected to sit an examination designed for general physicians. The new Paediatric Part 1 examination for the MRCP has changed the emphasis in revising for this hurdle. This book will hopefully provide relevant practice in answering questions specifically aimed at paediatric problems, both in clinical and basic science fields.

All the questions are novel and are supported by short explanatory notes where appropriate. We hope they are instrumental in launching new generations of paediatricians into clinical practice.

London 1996   A. P. W.
                                                    G. S.

1. Endocrinology

1.1 Precocious puberty:
A is more common in males
B may occur in primary hypothyroidism
C is associated with congenital adrenal hyperplasia
D is usually gonadotrophin independent in girls
E characteristically presents with isolated pubic hair development

1.2 Recognized causes of tall stature include:
A maternal diabetes mellitus
B Beckwith-Weidemann syndrome
C Klinefelter syndrome
D Sotos syndrome
E homocystinuria

1.3 Congenital adrenal hypoplasia:
A is usually inherited as an autosomal recessive condition
B is associated with gonadotrophin hypersecretion
C is diagnosed by the detection of an elevated plasma 17-hydroxyprogesterone level
D causes female sexual ambiguity
E results in salt wasting

1.4 Which of the following are characteristic features of congenital hypothyroidism:
A low birthweight
B exomphalos
C prolonged neonatal unconjugated hyperbilirubinaemia
D normal appearance
E goitre

1.5 The McCune-Albright syndrome:
A is associated with smooth contoured café-au-lait patches
B may occur together with hyperthyroidism
C results in pubertal delay
D may have skeletal manifestations
E is usually accompanied by delayed skeletal maturation

1.1
A	**False**
B	**True**
C	**True**
D	**False**
E	**False**

Precocious puberty is much more common in girls. In girls, the aetiology is usually gonadotrophin dependent and often idiopathic. Hypothyroidism may result in precocious puberty although there is, unusually, growth failure. Isolated pubic hair development is termed premature adrenarche. This is a normal variant. If this is associated with virilization or additional signs of puberty, it may be due to congenital adrenal hyperplasia.

1.2
A	**False**
B	**False**
C	**True**
D	**True**
E	**True**

Tall stature is usually familial. Syndromes including Marfan syndrome and the phenotypically similar homocystinuria are less common. Sotos syndrome features cerebral gigantism with mental retardation and phenotypic abnormalities. Hyperinsulinism (infant of a diabetic mother or Beckwith syndrome) results in a large infant. As insulin ceases to be a significant growth factor after 10 months of age, the affected individual does not become tall.

1.3
A	**False**
B	**False**
C	**False**
D	**False**
E	**True**

Whilst variants may exist, the typical inheritance pattern is X-linked. Cortisol and aldosterone deficiency occurs and salt wasting is usually apparent. An enzyme block is not apparent so there is no detectable elevation of 17-hydroxyprogesterone precursor. As there are no extra precursors to channel into the androgen pathway, there is no evidence of sexual ambiguity. Associated features include: gonadotrophin deficiency, icthyosis, sensorineural deafness and myopathy.

1.4
A	**False**
B	**False**
C	**True**
D	**True**
E	**False**

Only 5% of affected infants exhibit clinical signs within the first week of life hence the need for screening. Affected babies often weigh above 3.5 kg. Characteristic features when present include: umbilical herniae, prolonged neonatal jaundice and large posterior fontanelle. Goitres are rare as the most common aetiology remains athyreosis.

1.5
A	**False**
B	**True**
C	**False**
D	**True**
E	**False**

The McCune-Albright syndrome comprises ragged contoured café-au-lait patches, polyostotic fibrous dysplasia, precocious puberty (usually gonadotrophin independent) and hormonal hypersecretion. The 'bone age' is usually advanced along with the precocious puberty.

1.6 **Which of the following statements regarding growth hormone physiology are correct:**
   A secretion is pulsatile with a cycle of 180 minutes
   B growth hormone secretion is unaffected by somatostatin levels
   C is unaffected by insulin-like growth factor I secretion
   D is secreted from the anterior pituitary gland
   E is the main growth mediator in the first 6 months of life

1.7 **Which of the following are recognized causes of short stature:**
   A Laron syndrome
   B Mauriac syndrome
   C Russell-Silver syndrome
   D intrauterine growth retardation
   E Crohn's disease

1.8 **Macrocephaly may be a feature of:**
   A neurofibromatosis type I
   B Patau syndrome
   C oxycephaly
   D Dandy-Walker syndrome
   E Canavan's disease

1.9 **Congenital adrenal hyperplasia:**
   A is usually due to 21-hydroxylase deficiency
   B is associated with hypokalaemia in cases of 21-hydroxylase deficiency
   C always presents in the neonatal period
   D is a cause of primary amenorrhoea
   E may result in hypertension

1.6
A	**True**
B	**False**
C	**False**
D	**True**
E	**False**

Growth hormone, the main growth mediator after the first year of life, is secreted from the anterior pituitary in a pulsatile manner. The pulses are maintained by the interaction of somatostatin, growth hormone releasing hormone, other growth factors and cholinergic nerves. Disordered pulsatile secretion may cause growth failure in the absence of growth hormone deficiency due to gene deletion.

1.7
A	**True**
B	**True**
C	**True**
D	**True**
E	**True**

Many different conditions cause growth failure and subsequent short stature. Laron syndrome is a result of growth hormone receptor deficiency. Mauriac syndrome occurs in poorly controlled diabetics who exhibit poor growth and hepatomegaly. Intrauterine growth retardation (IUGR) may, in severe cases, cause short stature. The Russell-Silver syndrome is the association of severe IUGR short stature, somatic asymmetry, clinodactyly and, often, mild cognitive impairment. Short stature may be the only sign of Crohn's disease.

1.8
A	**True**
B	**False**
C	**False**
D	**True**
E	**True**

Macrocephaly is most commonly familial. Chromosomal anomalies tend to cause microcephaly, e.g. Patau syndrome. Some forms of craniosynostosis, e.g. oxycephaly, also cause microcephaly. Approximately 40% of those with neurofibromatosis have macrocephaly. Inherited metabolic disorders which cause the accumulation of abnormal cells result in increased brain mass (megalencephaly). These include Tay-Sachs disease and Canavan's disease. The Dandy-Walker syndrome is the association of cerebellar hypoplasia and a fourth ventricle cyst.

1.9
A	**True**
B	**False**
C	**False**
D	**True**
E	**True**

Adrenal hormone biosynthesis may be affected by many enzyme deficiencies. The most common is 21-hydroxylase deficiency. Females exhibit sexual ambiguity. Salt wasting occurs in two-thirds of sufferers. Whilst presentation is most common in the neonatal period, late onset disease may present with precocious puberty and amenorrhoea. Hyperkalaemia occurs in the most common salt wasting variant of 21-hydroxylase deficiency. Hypertension is a feature of the 11β-hydroxylase deficient variety.

1.10 Pubertal delay:
A is more common in males
B is associated with Turner syndrome
C may be familial
D does not affect height velocity
E growth hormone is the treatment of choice

1.11 Polycystic ovarian disease:
A may occur in treated congenital adrenal hyperplasia
B does not affect fertility
C causes precocious puberty
D is associated with menorrhagia
E is associated with clitoromegaly

1.12 The following are true of hormone binding proteins:
A insulin-like growth factors are the only hormones without specific binding proteins
B 30–50% of circulating growth hormone is bound to a binding protein
C growth hormone binding proteins are membrane bound receptors
D binding proteins are all variants of albumen
E lack of growth hormone binding protein results in Laron syndrome

1.13 When predicting future growth potential:
A both parents' heights may be plotted directly on the child's centile chart
B the child's expected height range is the sum of the parental heights
C the child's expected height range is independent of skeletal maturity
D the child's expected height range is more accurately assessed from measurements of 'sitting height'
E the child's expected height range is accurate in children with skeletal dysplasia

1.10	A	True	Pubertal delay is more common in males where it is usually constitutional in nature with a familial predilection. Girls may be affected by Turner syndrome. Delayed puberty also delays the pubertal growth spurt forcing the child to grow in a prepubertal manner with a decreasing height velocity until puberty ensues or is promoted. Growth hormone is of little practical use and the drugs of choice are anabolic or sex steroids.
	B	True	
	C	True	
	D	False	
	E	False	

1.11	A	True	Polycystic ovarian disease is a common cause of irregular menorrhagia, oligomenorrhoea and pubertal delay. Only some affected females exhibit hirsutism. Clitoromegaly is a feature of marked virilization and is absent in polycystic ovarian disease. Treated congenital adrenal hyperplasia may be associated with polycystic ovaries and therefore account for the degree of subfertility encountered in this condition.
	B	False	
	C	False	
	D	True	
	E	False	

1.12	A	False	Many hormones are bound to both albumen, globulin and also specific binding proteins. Insulin-like growth factors bind to a series of binding proteins as does growth hormone. The physiological function of this arrangement is still uncertain. Growth hormone binding proteins are believed to arise from either cleavage of the hormone receptor protein or by alternative splicing of receptor messenger RNA. Although a deficiency of growth hormone binding protein occurs in Laron syndrome, this is believed to be consequent upon a deficiency of the hormone receptor.
	B	True	
	C	False	
	D	False	
	E	False	

1.13	A	False	Prediction of final height is difficult. A correction factor of 12.5 cm is necessary when plotting the height of the other sex parent on their child's growth chart. This is added to a maternal height when plotting on her son's chart and subtracted from the paternal height when plotting on his daughter's centiles. The expected height range is 8 cm above and below the mid-parental height when the parental heights have been corrected. Skeletal maturity is important in height prediction except in cases of skeletal dysplasia where the skeletal bone age is unreliable. The 'sitting height' is of value in determining the presence of a skeletal dysplasia.
	B	False	
	C	False	
	D	False	
	E	False	

1.14 Cushing's disease:
A is associated with growth retardation
B is usually confirmed by measurement of a random cortisol level
C may be associated with hypocalcaemia
D is usually due to ectopic ACTH secretion
E may result in skin depigmentation

1.15 The following statements about pubertal status are true:
A an orchidometer testicular volume of 6 ml is prepubertal
B staging may be performed using the Tanner staging system
C the onset of female puberty occurs with breast development stage 2
D boys undergo an early pubertal growth spurt
E menarche is an early feature of female puberty

1.16 Features of juvenile hypothyroidism include:
A decreased sleep requirement
B increased hair growth
C poor school performance
D tremor
E delayed ankle reflex

1.17 The following are causes of sexual ambiguity:
A 5α-reductase deficiency
B XO/XY
C 17-hydroxylase deficiency congenital adrenal hyperplasia
D XXY
E XO mosaicism

1.14 A **True**   Cushing's disease is associated with growth
      B **False**   retardation, weight gain and abdominal striae.
      C **False**   Hypercalcaemia may occur. Hyperpigmentation
      D **False**   associated with ACTH excess occurs if this is the
      E **False**   underlying pathophysiology or associated with
                        adrenalectomy treatment (Nelson syndrome).
                        Hypercortisolism cannot be confirmed by an elevated
                        cortisol level.

1.15 A **False**   Whilst both sexes generally enter puberty within 6
      B **True**   months of each other, the sequence of pubertal
      C **True**   changes differs between sexes. Disordered pattern of
      D **False**   pubertal changes is termed dissonance and indicates
      E **False**   an endocrinopathy. Puberty may be assessed using
                        the Tanner staging system. Girls commence puberty
                        with breast development followed by an early growth
                        spurt. Menarche is a late feature of puberty. Boys
                        begin with testicular development as measured using
                        an orchidometer. A testicular volume of 4 ml indicates
                        the onset of puberty. The pubertal growth spurt is a
                        late feature of male puberty.

1.16 A **False**   Juvenile hypothyroidism is usually due to thyroiditis.
      B **False**   The onset is often insidious with a deterioration in
      C **True**   school performance. Cold intolerance, dry skin, poor
      D **False**   hair growth are all features. A delayed ankle reflex is
      E **True**   a common clinical feature. The other features de-
                        scribed indicate hyperthyroidism.

1.17 A **True**   Sexual ambiguity is, clinically, often a case of female
      B **True**   masculinization. In this situation the most common
      C **True**   cause is 21-hydroxylase congenital adrenal
      D **False**   hyperplasia. 17-hydroxylase prevents adrenal
      E **False**   androgen synthesis resulting in male
                        undermasculinization as a variant of congenital
                        adrenal hyperplasia. 5α-reductase deficiency is
                        another cause of male sexual ambiguity. This
                        hormone converts testosterone to the active
                        metabolite, dihydrotestosterone, which is important in
                        the virilization of the external male genitalia. XO/XY
                        results in a form of hermaphroditism (mixed gonadal
                        dysgenesis). XXY is Klinefelter syndrome with
                        phenotypic male appearance. XO mosaicism results
                        in Turner syndrome.

1.18 Which of the following statements regarding calcium and phosphorus metabolism are correct:
  A renal tubules can reabsorb only 5% of filtered calcium
  B parathyroid hormone action results in decreased intestinal absorption of calcium
  C renal phosphate excretion is stimulated by parathyroid hormone
  D calcitonin reduces serum phosphate levels
  E vitamin D stimulates intestinal absorption of calcium

1.19 Features of hypoparathyroidism include:
  A magnesium toxicity
  B metastatic calcification
  C choreiform movements
  D constipation
  E brachydactyly

1.20 Nephrogenic diabetes insipidus:
  A results from a deficiency of vasopressin
  B is an autosomal recessive condition
  C May cause severe hyponatraemia
  D is diagnosed by a water challenge test
  E is a feature of Wolfram syndrome

1.18 A **False** The following are the major actions of the various
     B **False** hormones involved in calcium/phosphorus
     C **True**   metabolism:
     D **True**   **Parathyroid hormone:** increases calcium levels by
     E **True**   stimulating bone release, increasing intestinal
                  absorption and increasing tubular reabsorption.
                  Phosphate renal clearance is increased.
                  Vitamin D: increases intestinal absorption of calcium,
                  mobilizes calcium from bone; improves renal
                  reabsorption of calcium; and increases phosphate
                  levels by enhancing intestinal and renal reabsorption.
                  Calcitonin: lowers serum calcium and inhibits bone
                  release; and lowers serum phosphate by decreasing
                  renal reabsorption.

1.19 A **False** Hypoparathyroidism causes hypocalcaemia. In
     B **True**   addition, raised intracranial pressure, hyperreflexia,
     C **True**   choreiform movements, metastatic calcification and
     D **False** gastrointestinal hyperactivity occur. Magnesium
     E **False** deficiency may coexist. Brachydactyly is a feature of
                  pseudohypoparathyroidism.

1.20 A **False** Nephrogenic diabetes insipidus is usually X-linked or
     B **False** more rarely an autosomal dominant inherited
     C **False** disorder. Hypernatraemia is a risk. The
     D **False** pathophysiology is renal unresponsiveness to
     E **True**   vasopressin. Diagnosis is via a failed water
                  deprivation test with no improvement after the
                  diagnostic administration of vasopressin. It is a
                  feature of Wolfram syndrome (DIDMOAD = diabetes
                  insipidus + diabetes mellitus + optic atrophy +
                  deafness).

2. Infections

2.1 **Human herpes virus type 6:**
  A causes erythema infectiosum
  B produces a marked atypical lymphocytosis
  C is neurotropic
  D results in a rash which commences behind the ears
  E causes a defervescent illness (rash appears as fever settles)

2.2 **Which of the following are consistent with the diagnosis of the toxic shock syndrome:**
  A normotension
  B core temperature of 36.5°C
  C elevated plasma creatine kinase
  D purpura
  E diarrhoea

2.3 **The following are recognized causes of congenital infection:**
  A parvovirus B19
  B HTLV1
  C coxsackie B viruses
  D varicella-zoster
  E *Toxocara canis*

2.4 **Which of the following infectious diseases are correctly matched with their incubation period:**
  A roseola infantum: 2–5 days
  B measles: 1–4 days
  C mumps: 7–10 days
  D varicella: 14–20 days
  E erythema infectiosum: 18–21 days

2.1	A	False	Human herpes virus type 6 (HHV6) is responsible for roseola infantum. Clinically, the febrile illness lasts for 3–5 days. The fever suddenly subsides on the appearance of the erythematous macular rash. This commences on the trunk. This typical illness only accounts for 17% of HHV6 infections. It is responsible for one-third of febrile convulsions in those under 2 years of age. Though neurotropic, HHV6 is rarely identified in CSF although viral nucleic acid may be detectable. Encephalopathy and thrombocytopenia are potential complications.
	B	False	
	C	True	
	D	False	
	E	True	

2.2	A	False	The toxic shock syndrome (TSS) has been documented with staphylococcal sepsis and also streptococcal and adenoviral infections. In staphylococcal TSS, a 22 kDa protein toxin is produced which nonspecifically activates lymphocytes in a polyclonal fashion. This is an example of a superantigen disorder. Clinical features include: fever of at least 38.9°C; generalized skin erythema with subsequent desquamation; hypotension and evidence of toxin action on three systems – diarrhoea/vomiting, myalgia or elevated creatine kinase, mucous membrane changes, thrombocytopenia and altered mental state.
	B	False	
	C	True	
	D	True	
	E	True	

2.3	A	True	Whilst the classic acronym TORCH cites some of the possible agents causing congenital infection, many more have also been implicated. Cytomegalovirus (CMV) remains the most common congenital infection in the UK. Varicella is a rare cause of embryopathy associated with circumferential limb scars and defects. Parvovirus infection in the second trimester may result in hydrops fetalis and fetal death. HIV infection can occur during pregnancy. HTLV1 and enteroviruses do not classically cause a congenital infection.
	B	False	
	C	True	
	D	True	
	E	False	

2.4	A	False	The following are the correct incubation periods: roseola infantum: 10–15 days measles: 10–14 days mumps: 14–28 days varicella: 7–21 days erythema infectiosum: 4–14 days
	B	False	
	C	False	
	D	True	
	E	False	

2.5 **Which of the following statements regarding transmission of HIV infection are correct:**
   A rate of vertical transmission in western Europe is 60%
   B transmission risk is increased when maternal CD4 lymphocyte counts are low
   C transmission through breast milk has not been recorded
   D zidovudine therapy in pregnancy does not affect transmission rates
   E persistence of anti-HIV IgG after 3 months of age is indicative of HIV infection

2.6 **Clinical features of Kawasaki's disease include:**
   A splenomegaly
   B acute non-calculous hydrops of the gallbladder
   C perineal accentuation of the polymorphous skin rash
   D coronary artery aneurysms
   E peripheral desquamation within the first week of fever

2.7 **Poor prognostic indicators in meningococcal septicaemia include:**
   A concomitant meningitis
   B peripheral neutrophil count of $24 \times 10^9/l$
   C male sex
   D age greater than 4 years
   E purpura present for 8 hours prior to treatment

2.8 **The following may be caused by adenovirus infection:**
   A febrile convulsion
   B toxic shock syndrome
   C bronchiolitis
   D pneumonia
   E keratoconjunctivitis

2.5   A False   Vertical transmission rates are 15–20% in Europe but
      B True   higher in Africa. Breast feeding doubles the risk.
      C False   Zidovudine may reduce the risk by 65%. Early
      D False   neonatal diagnosis is difficult as anti-HIV IgM is
      E False   unreliable but anti-HIV IgG may be maternal in origin.
                    However, persistence of this IgG after 18 months of
                    age indicates true infection. Other methods to confirm
                    infection earlier include: viral culture; detection of viral
                    nucleic acid; detection of viral antigen and viral
                    products.

2.6   A False   There is no diagnostic test for Kawasaki's disease.
      B True   Many cases do not fulfil all the accepted diagnostic
      C True   criteria. A mild obstructive hepatitis may occur and
      D True   non-calculous hydrops of the gallbladder occurs in
      E False   3%. The skin rash is polymorphous and may even
                    appear urticarial. Perineal accentuation often occurs.
                    Peripheral desquamation occurs in the second week.
                    Cardiovascular involvement occurs in 20–30% with
                    pancarditis or coronary artery aneurysm formation.
                    The median time for echocardiographic evidence is
                    10 days although they may form before this time.
                    Those less than 8 mm in diameter regress in 60% of
                    cases.

2.7   A False   Meningococcal septicaemia with profound shock has
      B False   a mortality of 30–40%. Increased risk factors include
      C True   young age, male sex, and overwhelming sepsis
      D False   without evidence of host response, i.e. lack of
      E True   peripheral neutrophilia. Delay in diagnosis or treat-
                    ment are adverse prognostic factors.

2.8   A True   Adenoviruses are non-encapsulated DNA containing
      B True   viruses. They account for 5–8% of paediatric
      C True   respiratory infections. A severe bronchiolitic illness
      D True   may occur resulting in destructive lung disease.
      E True   Adenoviruses may cause 10% of childhood
                    pneumonias. Together with HHV6, adenoviruses are
                    often precipitants of febrile convulsions.

2.9 In typhoid:
 A there is an incubation period of 14–21 days
 B reliable detection is by the Widal serological test
 C diagnosis may be by the development of 'rose spots' after 48 hours
 D stool culture is most commonly positive in the first week of the illness
 E chronic carriage may be eradicated by ciprofloxacin

2.10 Recognized features of the haemolytic-uraemic syndrome include:
 A thrombocytopenia
 B winter seasonal predominance
 C bloody diarrhoea prodrome in over 60% of affected children
 D verocytotoxin producing *Escherichia coli* serotype 0157
 E renal failure

2.11 Patients with the Hyper-IgE syndrome:
 A suffer recurrent viral infections
 B have low CD4 peripheral lymphocyte counts
 C have a marked basophilia
 D may develop pneumatoceles
 E may respond to histamine H_2-receptor antagonists

2.12 Which of the following are examples of 'superantigen' disorders:
 A staphylococcal toxic shock syndrome
 B haemorrhagic shock and encephalopathy syndrome
 C cat-scratch disease
 D neonatal scalded skin syndrome
 E Creutzfeldt-Jakob disease

2.9 A **True**   Typhoid fever, caused by *Salmonella typhi*, has an
     B **False**   incubation period of 7–21 days. Constipation is
     C **False**   common although diarrhoea may occur in the second
     D **False**   week. Classically there is a fever without a coexisting
     E **True**   tachycardia. Sparse erythematous macules ('rose
                    spots') may appear on the trunk about the tenth day.
                    Complications include: splenomegaly; gastrointestinal
                    haemorrhage and perforation; hepatitis; and
                    depression. Blood cultures are usually positive in the
                    first week and stool cultures in the second. Culture
                    has superseded the unreliable Widal serological test.

2.10 A **True**   Verotoxigenic *Escherichia coli* O157 is the usual agent
     B **False**   causing the haemolytic-uraemic syndrome. Toxin-
     C **True**   producing shigellae have also been documented as
     D **True**   aetiological agents. There is a peak incidence in July
     E **True**   and August. Oligaemia and acute renal failure follow a
                    bout of bloody diarrhoea. The incubation period is 2–7
                    days. Treatment is supportive.

2.11 A **False**   The immunodeficiency Hyper-IgE syndrome presents
     B **False**   with recurrent abscess formation. Respiratory
     C **False**   staphylococcal infections may cause pneumatoceles.
     D **True**   Patchy dermatitis occurs. The inheritance is
     E **True**   autosomal dominant with variable penetrance. An
                    eosinophilia of 50–60% may occur but the lymphocyte
                    counts are normal. Whilst the IgE levels are greatly
                    elevated, the other immunoglobulins are either low or
                    normal. Treatment includes antibiotics and the use of
                    H_2-receptor blockers, e.g. cimetidine.

2.12 A **True**   A superantigen is a peptide antigen (often a bacterial
     B **False**   toxin) which can nonspecifically polyclonally stimulate
     C **False**   a large number of lymphocytes. These superantigens
     D **True**   do not need to fit into a specific receptor site to
     E **False**   stimulate the lymphocyte but can bind to various
                    receptors. Examples include staphylococcal toxic
                    shock syndrome and the neonatal scalded skin
                    syndrome. Cat-scratch disease is a bacterial infection
                    with the Gram-negative bacillus *Rochalimaea
                    henselae*. Creutzfeldt-Jakob disease is a prion
                    disorder. The cause of the haemorrhagic shock and
                    encephalopathy syndrome is still uncertain.

2.13 **Characteristic features of Familial Mediterranean Fever include:**
 A peritonitis
 B arthritis
 C amyloidosis
 D autosomal dominant inheritance
 E pleurisy

2.14 **Which of the following are examples of rickettsial infections:**
 A roseola infantum
 B ehrlichiosis
 C typhus
 D anthrax
 E plague

2.15 **Which of the statements regarding infectious mononucleosis are correct:**
 A severe airway obstruction is resistant to steroid therapy
 B heterophile antibodies are Epstein-Barr virus (EBV) specific
 C the Paul-Bunnell test is positive in 90% of childhood infections
 D the incubation period is 2–5 days
 E splenomegaly occurs in 2% of cases

2.16 **Molluscum contagiosum infection:**
 A typically appears on the palms and soles
 B is a fungal infection
 C is self-limiting
 D manifests as pedunculated papules
 E characteristically occurs in the buccal cavity

2.17 **Which of the following infections are correctly paired with their characteristic skin rash:**
 A Lyme disease: erythema marginatum
 B parvovirus 19: erythema chronicum migrans
 C tuberculosis: erythema nodosum
 D syphilis: erythema ab igne
 E *Mycoplasma pneumoniae*: erythema multiforme

2.13 A **True** Familial Mediterranean fever (FMF), an autosomal
     B **True** recessive disorder, causes periodic fever associated
     C **True** with polyserositis. A higher incidence occurs in
     D **False** Mediterranean races and some Jewish groups. There
     E **True** is no diagnostic test. Systemic amyloidosis often
                 resulting in renal failure remains the most frequent
                 complication. Colchicine is an effective treatment.

2.14 A **False** Ehrlichiosis is an acute febrile rickettsial illness. It
     B **True** resembles Rocky Mountain spotted fever.
     C **True** Tetracyclines are the treatment of choice. Roseola is
     D **False** caused by HHV6. Anthrax and plague are bacterial
     E **False** infections. The former may be cutaneous, pneumonic
                 or enteric. The pneumonic type of anthrax has a high
                 mortality. The antibiotic of choice is penicillin.

2.15 A **False** Infectious mononucleosis due to the Epstein-Barr
     B **False** virus (EBV) may cause severe upper airway
     C **False** obstruction which responds dramatically to steroids.
     D **False** The heterophile antibodies are non-specific and are
     E **False** utilized in the Monospot and Paul-Bunnell screening
                 tests. They agglutinate horse and sheep erythrocytes
                 respectively. These tests are negative in about 50%
                 of paediatric infections. EBV has an incubation period
                 of 10–50 days. Splenomegaly occurs in 50% and
                 hepatitis in 10–15% of sufferers.

2.16 A **False** Molluscum contagiosum is caused by a DNA virus.
     B **False** The lesions appear as umbilicated papules. The
     C **True** palms and soles of the feet are usually spared and
     D **False** intraoral lesions are rare. The crushed and stained
     E **False** contents of a papule show the typical intracytoplasmic
                 bodies (Henderson-Patterson bodies).

2.17 A **False** Lyme disease is associated with erythema chronicum
     B **False** migrans whereas erythema marginatum is a feature
     C **True** of rheumatic fever. Parvovirus B19 infection appears
     D **False** as the 'slapped cheek' syndrome. Various skin
     E **True** manifestations accompany mycoplasma infection
                 including erythema multiforme. Erythema ab igne
                 results from thermal trauma.

2.18 **Human parvovirus B19 infection may cause:**
 A exanthema subitum
 B arthralgia
 C bullous myringitis
 D hydrops fetalis
 E aplastic anaemia in chronic haemolytic states

2.19 **Which of the following are 'major' criteria in the diagnosis of rheumatic fever:**
 A first degree heart block
 B arthralgia
 C recent streptococcal infection
 D Heberden's nodes
 E Sydenham's chorea

2.20 **Contraindications to performing a lumbar puncture in cases of suspected meningococcal meningitis include:**
 A Glasgow Coma Score of 4
 B unilateral fixed dilated pupil
 C petechial rash
 D cerebral confusion
 E palpably full anterior fontanelle

2.21 **Mumps infection:**
 A is always bilateral
 B is infectious until 1 day after the appearance of the parotid swelling
 C is the only cause of viral sialadenitis
 D may cause meningoencephalitis
 E responds to acyclovir

2.18 A **False**   Human parvovirus B19 infection is spread mainly by
      B **True**   droplets and has an incubation period of 4–14 days.
      C **False**   The typical lacy reticular rash associated with
      D **True**   reddened cheeks is termed erythema infectiosum or
      E **True**   fifth disease. Asymptomatic infection is common
                       (20%). This virus is also responsible for arthralgia,
                       aplastic crises in those with chronic haemolytic
                       disorders and fetal infection. Bullous myringitis is due
                       to mycoplasma infection.

2.19 A **False**   The revised MAJOR criteria are:
      B **False**   • flitting polyarthritis
      C **False**   • carditis
      D **False**   • Sydenham's chorea
      E **True**   • erythema marginatum
                       • subcutaneous nodules
                       MINOR criteria include:
                       • evidence of streptococcal disease
                       • arthralgia
                       • fever
                       • elevated acute phase reactants
                       • prolonged PR interval on ECG

2.20 A **True**   Lumbar puncture may be hazardous in patients
      B **True**   suffering raised intracranial pressure, septicaemia
      C **True**   with deranged coagulation or those who have
      D **True**   precarious respiratory function. A full anterior
      E **False**   fontanelle does indicate some intracranial
                       hypertension although the risk of coning is
                       substantially reduced by the open state of the
                       fontanelle.

2.21 A **False**   Mumps, caused by a myxovirus, is the most common
      B **False**   viral sialadenitis. Enteroviruses, parainfluenzae and
      C **False**   HIV viruses have also been documented. Mumps
      D **True**   infectivity lasts from the onset of parotid swelling until
      E **False**   complete resolution. The gland involvement may be
                       either unilateral or bilateral covering the preauricular
                       region to the angle of the jaw. The illness lasts for a
                       week. Complications include meningoencephalitis,
                       deafness, pancreatitis, oophoritis and orchitis.

2.22 Chronic granulomatous disease:
A results in recurrent viral infections
B has a multifactorial inheritance
C results from a defect in T cell activation
D may be complicated by pulmonary aspergillosis
E may be diagnosed using the nitroblue tetrazolium reduction test

2.23 Visceral leishmaniasis:
A causes hepatomegaly without splenomegaly
B results from parasitic invasion of the reticuloendothelial system
C has a 2–6 week incubation period
D is diagnosed on blood culture
E is transmitted by sandflies

2.24 Which of the following are recognized complications of varicella infection:
A massive skin necrosis
B orchitis
C Reye syndrome
D pneumonitis
E acute cerebellar ataxia

2.25 Which of the following disorders are caused by streptococcus:
A Kawasaki's disease
B scarlet fever
C glomerulonephritis
D necrotizing fasciitis
E Vincent's angina

2.22 A **False**   An X-linked inheritance occurs in 75% of cases of
      B **False**   chronic granulomatous disease. The basic defect of
      C **False**   immunity is monocyte oxidative killing. The nitroblue
      D **True**   tetrazolium test (NBT) is the screening test. Chronic
      E **True**   deep infections occur. Aspergillosis is a common
                    secondary pathogen.

2.23 A **False**   Visceral leishmaniasis (kala-azar) is transmitted by
      B **True**   sandflies. The incubation period is usually 3–8
      C **False**   months although it may be up to 10 years. Massive
      D **False**   hepatosplenomegaly occurs with anaemia and
      E **True**   lymphadenopathy. Demonstration of the parasite in
                    bone marrow or visceral biopsy remains the main
                    diagnostic technique. The cause of death is often
                    secondary infection.

2.24 A **True**   Varicella infection may be severe in adults particularly
      B **False**   pregnant women. Pneumonitis affecting varicella
      C **True**   during pregnancy has a mortality of 40%. Massive
      D **True**   skin necrosis may occur as part of a generalized
      E **True**   coagulopathy associated with transient autoantibody
                    induced protein C deficiency. Acute cerebellar
                    ataxia is a common complication during
                    convalescence with recovery the norm. Reye
                    syndrome has been documented after varicella
                    infection.

2.25 A **False**   Exotoxin producing strains of Group A β-haemolytic
      B **True**   streptococci cause scarlet fever. The cause of
      C **True**   Kawasaki's disease is uncertain although some
      D **True**   authorities believe it to be due to a superantigen
      E **False**   disorder. The superantigen may be a toxin produced
                    by the staphylococci. Vincent's angina is caused by a
                    Borrelia infection.

3. Neonatology

3.1 Recognized causes of the 'floppy baby' include:
 A trisomy 21
 B Zellweger syndrome
 C Becker muscular dystrophy
 D spinal muscular atrophy
 E hypothyroidism

3.2 Which of the following may cause apnoea in preterm infants:
 A hypocalcaemia
 B hypoglycaemia
 C respiratory syncytial virus infection
 D caffeine
 E intraventricular haemorrhage

3.3 Failure of resuscitation of a newborn may be due to:
 A patent ductus arteriosus
 B ventriculoseptal defect
 C congenital diaphragmatic hernia
 D pulmonary hypoplasia
 E hyaline membrane disease

3.4 Features of intrauterine growth retardation include:
 A neutropenia
 B hypoglycaemia
 C necrotizing enterocolitis
 D weight loss exceeding 10% of birthweight in first week
 E thermal instability

3.1	A	**True**	There are many causes of neonatal 'floppiness'.
	B	**True**	These may be divided into paralytic and non-paralytic
	C	**False**	disorders. This distinction may be made by the infant
	D	**True**	moving against gravity or maintaining position of a
	E	**True**	passively elevated limb. Paralytic disorders include spinal muscular atrophy, myopathies and other neuromuscular problems. Non-paralytic disorders include: CNS problems including trauma, asphyxia and chromosomal/syndromic conditions, connective tissue disorders and metabolic problems. The age of onset of Becker dystrophy is not neonatal.
3.2	A	**True**	Apnoea is common. Often the cause is prematurity
	B	**True**	although there are many pathological causes
	C	**True**	including metabolic and neurological disturbances.
	D	**False**	RSV infection may present with apnoea. Caffeine acts
	E	**True**	as a respiratory stimulant.
3.3	A	**False**	Failure to resuscitate may be due to lung problems
	B	**False**	(hypoplasia, pneumothorax or abnormal lung),
	C	**True**	mechanical problems (blockage of an endotracheal
	D	**True**	tube), overwhelming intrapartum sepsis or CNS
	E	**False**	catastrophe. Hyaline membrane disease develops postnatally. Cardiac lesions with obstruction to the right outflow tract with duct dependent circulation may rarely result in this situation.
3.4	A	**True**	Intrauterine growth retardation causes fetal stress.
	B	**True**	Transient haematological features include
	C	**True**	thrombocytopenia and neutropenia. Poor glycogen
	D	**False**	stores expose the infant to the risk of hypoglycaemia.
	E	**True**	Poor mesenteric blood flow may affect the gut mucosa and thus place the neonate at risk of necrotizing enterocolitis. The large surface area to body mass results in thermal instability. These infants do not usually lose weight in the first week provided they receive appropriate nutrition.

3.5 **Which of the following statements regarding surfactant therapy is correct:**
A the incidence of pneumothorax is reduced
B the incidence of intraventricular haemorrhage is reduced
C early therapy (within 4 hours) is more beneficial than later administration (after 12 hours)
D prolonged courses of surfactant therapy confer advantages
E the incidence of chronic lung disease is increased

3.6 **Which of the following statements regarding periventricular haemorrhage are correct:**
A most haemorrhages occur after the fourth day of life
B over 80% of haemorrhages progress to ventricular dilatation
C most cases of posthaemorrhagic hydrocephalus are communicating
D early ventricular tapping improves neurological outcome
E haemorrhage is usually caused by hypoglycaemia

3.7 **Recognized therapy for chronic neonatal lung disease include:**
A surfactant
B inhaled steroids
C chlorthiazide
D salbutamol
E vitamin E

3.8 **Risk factors for the development of necrotizing enterocolitis include:**
A fetal hyperechogenic gut on antenatal ultrasonography
B patent ductus arteriosus
C breast milk
D indomethacin therapy
E umbilical arterial catheter

3.5 A **True**   Most trials of various surfactants have shown a
     B **True**   reduction in the incidence of pneumothorax.
     C **True**   Intraventricular haemorrhage is also reduced in the
     D **False**   majority of studies although one study revealed the
     E **False**   reverse. The OSIRIS collaborative study
                     demonstrated benefits from early administration of
                     surfactant but prolonged dosage was no more
                     beneficial than the standard two doses 12 hours
                     apart. No consistent effect on chronic lung disease
                     has been demonstrated.

3.6 A **False**   Periventricular haemorrhage usually occurs within the
     B **False**   first 72 hours. Only the severe Grade 3 and 4
     C **True**   haemorrhages usually progress to posthaemorrhagic
     D **False**   ventricular dilatation which is most commonly
     E **False**   communicating with a block at the level of the
                     arachnoid granulations. Haemorrhage may be
                     precipitated by many adverse events particularly
                     pneumothorax and changes in cerebral blood flow.
                     Hypoglycaemia is not a common cause of PVH.
                     Studies have shown that there is no neurological
                     benefit from CSF removal by ventricular taps.

3.7 A **False**   Therapy for chronic lung disease is still controversial.
     B **True**   Dexamethasone has been shown to reduce ventilator
     C **True**   dependency but not oxygen dependency. Inhaled
     D **True**   steroids are currently under study and appear
     E **False**   efficacious. Diuretics have beneficial effects both by
                     their diuretic effect and by the effect on diaphragmatic
                     function. In some infants, salbutamol has a definite
                     effect, particularly in reducing airway obstruction.

3.8 A **True**   The pathophysiology of necrotizing enterocolitis is
     B **True**   complex and the aetiology is multifactorial.
     C **False**   Disturbance to mesenteric blood flow due to
     D **True**   catheters, drugs (indomethacin) or abnormal flow
     E **True**   (PDA) is often implicated. Antenatal gut ischaemia
                     may be detected by the ultrasound image of fetal
                     hyperechogenic gut. Breast milk has some protective
                     effects.

Neonatology

3.9 Criteria used in the Apgar score include:
A core temperature
B heart rate
C respiratory rate
D skin thickness
E muscle tone

3.10 Characteristic features of neonatal abstinence syndrome include:
A sweating
B coughing
C sneezing
D tremor
E hyperphagia

3.11 Complications of phototherapy include:
A diarrhoea
B erythematous rash
C hyponatraemia
D skin discoloration
E peripheral desquamation

3.12 Classical clinical features indicative of necrotizing enterocolitis include:
A abdominal distension
B apnoea
C alkalosis
D bilious nasogastric aspirates
E hypotension

3.13 The preterm infant is at increased risk of:
A retinopathy
B meconium aspiration
C pulmonary haemorrhage
D phosphate deficiency
E jaundice

3.14 Which of the following are characteristic haemodynamic changes encountered at birth:
A increased pulmonary vascular pressure
B right to left flow through the ductus arteriosus
C closure of the ductus venosus
D increased right ventricular end diastolic pressure
E reversal of flow across the foramen ovale

3.9   A False   Whilst important, core temperature is not a feature of
      B True   the Apgar score. Skin thickness (texture) is a feature
      C True   of the Dubowitz score used in the assessment of
      D False   gestational age.
      E True

3.10 A True   Neonatal abstinence syndrome occurs in infants who
      B False   are undergoing withdrawal from maternal drug
      C True   misuse. Irritability is the key feature of opiate
      D False   withdrawal which may result in seizures. Non-opiates
      E True   may cause effects such as cerebral infarction but not
                   necessarily abstinence symptoms.

3.11 A True   Phototherapy may cause a photosensitivity rash and
      B True   diarrhoea. The latter may result in dehydration but
      C False   rarely electrolyte abnormalities. Skin discoloration
      D True   occurs following incorrect phototherapy for a
      E False   conjugated rather than an unconjugated
                   hyperbilirubinaemia.

3.12 A True   The clinical manifestation and subsequent
      B True   deterioration may be variable and often rapid.
      C False   Unrecognized NEC may result in shock, acidosis and
      D True   death.
      E True

3.13 A True   The preterm infant does not usually produce
      B False   meconium antenatally except in rare occurrence of
      C True   listeriosis. Pulmonary haemorrhage may occur after
      D True   surfactant therapy. Phosphate deficiency is one of the
      E True   features resulting in metabolic bone disease of
                   prematurity.

3.14 A False   Haemodynamic changes at birth include decrease in
      B False   pulmonary vascular pressure with changes in right
      C True   ventricular pressure, and reversal of flow left to right
      D False   across the ductus arteriosus. The foramen ovale
      E False   closes.

3.15 Features of polycythaemia include:
A increased viscosity above a threshold haematocrit of 0.85
B renal vein thrombosis
C hypocalcaemia
D hyperbilirubinaemia
E tachypnoea

3.16 Which of the following ventilator manipulations will improve hypoxia:
A reduction in peak inspiratory pressure
B reduction in positive end expiratory pressure
C increased inspiratory time
D artificial paralysis
E increased ventilator rate

3.17 Recognized features of hypoxic-ischaemic encephalopathy include:
A hyperphagia
B seizure
C abdominal distension
D irritability
E adductor spasm

3.18 Characteristics of neonatal metabolic bone disease include:
A hyperphosphataemia
B elevated alkaline phosphatase level by 7 days of age
C ventilator dependency
D apnoea
E pathological fractures

3.15 A **False** The hyperviscosity syndrome manifests as jitteriness
     B **True** and a propensity to thromboses, and intravascular
     C **True** sludging occurs with polycythaemia. The blood
     D **True** viscosity increases exponentially after a haematocrit
     E **True** of 0.60. Tachypnoea is a feature of the respiratory
                 problems of hyperviscosity. Polycythaemia results in
                 hypoglycaemia, hypocalcaemia and
                 hyperbilirubinaemia.

3.16 A **False** Oxygenation is proportional to the mean airway
     B **False** pressure (MAP). The MAP is increased by changes in
     C **True** the peak inspiratory pressure, end expiratory
     D **True** pressure and inspiratory time. If the infant is actively
     E **False** expiring against the inspiratory drive of the ventilator
                 then artificial paralysis will allow more efficient
                 ventilation and subsequent reduction in hypoxia.
                 Faster ventilatory rates are more useful in reducing
                 hypercarbia although there will be some minor
                 improvement in MAP.

3.17 A **False** Hypoxic-ischaemic encephalopathy (HIE) is often the
     B **True** result of a perinatal asphyxial insult. Mild symptoms
     C **False** are irritability with an abnormal high-pitched cry.
     D **True** Moderate symptoms include irritability and difficulty in
     E **False** feeding. Severe HIE results in seizures, raised
                 intracranial pressure and is often associated with
                 multisystem failure. Neonatal hyperphagia is a feature
                 of some abstinence syndromes. Adductor spasm is
                 often seen later in infants with a spastic diplegia.

3.18 A **False** Neonatal metabolic bone disease usually occurs in
     B **False** the smallest of infants after the first few weeks of life.
     C **True** The underlying problem seems to be substrate
     D **False** deficiency, particularly of phosphate.
     E **True** Hypophosphataemia should be avoided and
                 elevations of the serum alkaline phosphatase levels
                 are useful biochemical indices. Severe disease may
                 result in rickets, ventilator dependency due to thoracic
                 weakness and pathological fractures after trivial or
                 unrecognized trauma.

3.19 Causes of large-for-dates infants include:
A   Beckwith syndrome
B   growth hormone secreting adenoma
C   hypothyroidism
D   infant of a diabetic mother
E   Patau syndrome

3.20 Risk factors for the development of retinopathy include:
A   asphyxia
B   intrauterine growth retardation
C   prematurity
D   sepsis
E   oxygen administration

3.21 Refractory hypoxia may be caused by:
A   pulmonary hypertension
B   cyanotic cardiac disease
C   inappropriate ventilator settings
D   pulmonary interstitial emphysema
E   chronic lung disease

3.22 Which of the following maternal illnesses may cause neonatal disease:
A   systemic lupus erythematosus
B   mumps
C   lithium therapy
D   thyrotoxicosis
E   idiopathic thrombocytopenia

3.23 Which of the following statements regarding neonatal renal physiology are correct:
A   glomerular filtration rate is low at birth
B   plasma creatinine levels at delivery reflect renal function
C   plasma urea concentration reliably indicates renal function
D   urinary concentrating ability is greater than a normal adult
E   responsiveness to vasopressin is greater in preterm than term infants

3.19 A **True** Fetal growth is largely under the control of nutritional
      B **False** factors and nutritionally derived growth factors. Thus
      C **False** excessive fetal growth is due to such factors. This is
      D **True** often due to hyperinsulinaemia (infant of a diabetic
      E **False** mother; Beckwith syndrome). Growth hormone and
                   thyroid hormones are less important for the first 9
                   months of postnatal life. Patau syndrome often results
                   in growth retarded size.

3.20 A **False** Retinopathy of prematurity results from vascular
      B **True** proliferation in an immature eye. Low birth weight,
      C **True** preterm gestation and overall severity of illness are
      D **True** the major predictive factors. Retinopathy usually
      E **True** occurs 5 to 8 weeks after delivery. Oxygen
                   administration is also a risk factor.

3.21 A **True** Refractory hypoxia occurs either as a result of
      B **True** mechanical interference, e.g. inappropriate ventilation
      C **True** or mixing of oxygenated and deoxygenated blood by
      D **False** right to left circulatory flow. This may be due to a
      E **False** cyanotic lesion or by persistent fetal circulation as a
                   consequence of pulmonary hypertension.

3.22 A **True** Maternal SLE may be complicated by anti Ro
      B **True** antibodies which may induce fetal and neonatal heart
      C **True** block. Maternal mumps infection has resulted in fetal
      D **True** endocardial fibroelastosis. Lithium medication has
      E **True** been associated with embryopathy, particularly the
                   development of Ebstein's cardiac anomaly. Neonatal
                   thyrotoxicosis may be induced by the passage of
                   stimulatory IgG autoantibodies. Idiopathic
                   thrombocytopenia may result in transient neonatal
                   thrombocytopenia.

3.23 A **True** The glomerular filtration rate (GFR) and renal blood
      B **False** flow is low at birth but increases over the first 3 days
      C **False** of life. The GFR then increases as a function of
      D **False** postconceptual age. Birth creatinine levels reflect
      E **False** maternal levels and urea is not a reliable indicator of
                   renal function being dependent on catabolism and
                   muscle bulk. Renal tubular function is immature and
                   there is a reduced responsiveness to vasopressin.

3.24 Which of the following are adverse effects of cold stress:
A persistent fetal circulation
B hypovolaemia
C increased oxygen consumption
D increased surfactant production
E acidosis

3.25 Features suggestive of a tracheo-oesophageal fistula with oesophageal atresia include:
A failure to thrive
B recurrent pneumonia
C oliogohydramnios
D large amount of mucus in the pharynx at delivery
E slow to establish feeds

3.26 Which of the following metabolic disorders usually present in the neonatal period:
A non-ketotic hyperglycinaemia
B maple syrup urine disease
C Niemann-Pick disease
D isovaleric aciduria
E peroxisomal disorders

3.27 Periventricular leucomalacia:
A results from venous infarction
B occurs within 5 days of delivery
C is an indication for withdrawal of intensive support
D usually communicates with the ventricular system
E may be associated with visual loss

3.24 A **True**   Cold stress exacerbates any neonatal problems by
      B **True**   increasing both oxygen and glucose consumption.
      C **True**   Hypovolaemia may occur which leads to acidosis.
      D **False**   Surfactant production is impaired leading to a
      E **True**   worsening of respiratory function.

3.25 A **False**   Oesophageal atresia with coexisting fistula presents
      B **False**   early after or at delivery. Antenatally there may be a
      C **False**   history of polyhydramnios and indeed there may be a
      D **True**   large volume of mucus present in the pharynx at
      E **False**   delivery. Such children must not be fed until
                        oesophageal atresia has been actively excluded or
                        else there is a real risk of aspiration.

3.26 A **True**   Many different metabolic disorders may present in the
      B **True**   neonatal period. The usual manifestation is either
      C **False**   neurological (seizures; apnoea), infection, liver
      D **True**   failure, hypoglycaemia or acid/base disturbance. Non-
      E **True**   ketotic hyperglycinaemia is a cause of hiccoughs and
                        then neurological deterioration. Amino and organic
                        acidurias may present with various combinations of
                        the above. Peroxisomal disorders may show clinical
                        features within the neonatal period. Lysosomal
                        disorders more commonly present in infancy.

3.27 A **False**   Periventricular leucomalacia (PVL) arises from
      B **False**   ischaemic damage. Except for rare antenatal
      C **False**   examples, most cases manifest after 14 days. The
      D **False**   cysts may coalesce but do not usually connect with
      E **True**   the ventricular system unlike porencephalic cysts.
                        The latter usually occur after venous infarction.
                        Occipital PVL may result in visual impairment. The
                        prognosis is guarded but PVL is usually not an
                        indication for withdrawal of intensive care except
                        when severe, bilateral and in the parieto-occipital
                        region. This remains controversial.

3.28 Features of the normal preterm infant blood count include:
- A platelet count of 80 x 10^9/l
- B haematocrit of 0.30
- C lymphocytosis
- D mean corpuscular volume above 100 fl
- E absence of nucleated red blood cells

3.29 The development of pneumothorax is associated with:
- A surfactant therapy
- B artificial paralysis
- C patient triggered ventilation
- D meconium aspiration
- E pulmonary interstitial emphysema

3.30 Causes of neonatal vomiting include:
- A congenital adrenal hyperplasia
- B gastro-oesophageal reflux
- C subdural haemorrhage
- D urinary tract infection
- E metabolic disease

3.28 A **False**   The neonatal blood count differs from the adult or
      B **False**   older child. Erythrocytes are larger (greater MCV) and
      C **False**   the haemoglobin level is higher. Relative
      D **True**   polycythaemia occurs with the haematocrit
      E **False**   approximately 0.50. A level of 0.30 indicates anaemia,
                        usually due to blood loss and is an indication for
                        transfusion. The white count is often high and is
                        usually a neutrophilia. This then changes to a
                        lymphocyte predominance over the next few weeks.
                        Nucleated red cells are common. The platelet count
                        does not differ in the neonate compared to the adult
                        range.

3.29 A **False**   Pneumothorax often complicates ventilation in babies
      B **False**   with severe lung disease or those requiring high
      C **False**   inspiratory pressures. This is very apparent in cases
      D **True**   of meconium aspiration. Furthermore, asynchronous
      E **True**   ventilation is a risk factor which may be reduced by
                        artificial paralysis or patient triggered ventilation. In
                        some cases, pulmonary interstitial emphysema
                        precedes pneumothorax as the first sign of air leak.

3.30 A **True**   The causes are legion! They encompass gastro-
      B **True**   intestinal, endocrine, neurological, renal and meta-
      C **True**   bolic causes.
      D **True**
      E **True**

4. Development

4.1 Which of the following are primitive neonatal reflexes:
    A Moro reflex
    B sucking reflex
    C rooting reflex
    D gastrocolic reflex
    E Babinski reflex

4.2 A normal 9-month-old can
    A build a tower of 4 blocks
    B roll from supine to prone
    C weight bear
    D say 'mama' and 'dada'
    E wave bye-bye

4.3 A normal child can pick up objects
    A with a pincer grasp at 6 months
    B with a palmar grasp at 9 months
    C with a tripod grasp at 3 months
    D by reaching out to objects out of range by 3 months
    E and cast them at 1 year

4.4 A normal 2-year-old can
    A walk up stairs one step at a time
    B jump
    C hop on one leg
    D copy a circle
    E dress him/herself

4.5 Which of the following may indicate an underlying developmental problem:
    A unilateral Moro response
    B inability to walk at 20 months
    C inability to sit unsupported at 15 months
    D head lag present at 10 months of age
    E left handed preference at 6 months

4.1
A True
B True
C True
D False
E False

4.2
A False
B True
C True
D False
E False

The ability to build a tower of 4 cubes is attained at approximately 18 months. Verbal ability to use the words 'mama' and 'dada' occurs around 1 year as does the ability to wave bye-bye.

4.3
A False
B False
C False
D False
E True

The following are the ages for various grasps:
palmar: 6 months
tripod: 9 months
pincer: 1 year

4.4
A True
B True
C False
D False
E True

4.5
A True
B True
C True
D True
E True

A unilateral Moro reflex is associated with abnormalities including brachial plexus injury, cerebral palsy and pseudoparalysis such as a clavicular fracture. Failure to sit at 6–9 months and inability to walk by 18 months are worrying features. Hand preference should not be apparent within the first year.

5. Immunizations

5.1 Current contraindications to pertussis immunization include:
   A egg allergy
   B personal history of febrile convulsion
   C family history of epilepsy
   D indurated swelling following previous immunization
   E prolonged inconsolable crying for more than 4 hours with previous vaccination

5.2 Which of the following statements concerning the BCG vaccination are correct:
   A the vaccination must be given intradermally
   B the optimal site of vaccination is the insertion of the deltoid muscle near the middle of the upper arm
   C it is a protein derivative vaccine
   D it is contraindicated in children who are HIV positive
   E it has a protective efficacy of 95%

5.3 Which of the following are general contraindications to vaccination:
   A prematurity
   B cerebral palsy
   C eczema
   D history of neonatal jaundice
   E steroid therapy for congenital adrenal hyperplasia

5.4 The following vaccinations are contraindicated in HIV positive children:
   A measles
   B pertussis
   C hepatitis B
   D oral polio
   E *Haemophilus influenzae* type b (Hib)

5.1 A **False**   Current contraindications include: acute febrile
     B **False**   illness; previous severe local or generalized reaction
     C **False**   to pertussis vaccination including inconsolable crying,
     D **True**   anaphylaxis, unresponsiveness and convulsions
     E **True**   within 72 hours.

5.2 A **True**   The BCG is a live attenuated vaccine with an efficacy
     B **True**   of approximately 70%. Most complications
     C **False**   accompany incorrect vaccination technique. It must
     D **True**   be given intradermally. It is not to be given to children
     E **False**   known to be HIV positive.

5.3 A **False**   All these are oft quoted but inaccurate 'false'
     B **False**   contraindications. Replacement steroid therapy is not
     C **False**   a contraindication.
     D **False**
     E **False**

5.4 A **False**   Symptomatic HIV children may receive inactivated
     B **False**   oral polio or standard polio vaccine. They should not
     C **False**   receive BCG or yellow fever vaccines. Vaccine
     D **False**   efficacy may be reduced.
     E **False**

5.5 The Hib vaccine:
A has reduced the incidence of acute epiglottitis
B is a live vaccine
C is given as a booster vaccination at school entry
D protects against non-encapsulated haemophilus species
E primary course comprises three doses separated by 1 month

5.6 Varicella-zoster immunoglobulin:
A has a specific antibody content similar to standard immunoglobulin
B should be given to infants whose mothers have zoster infections
C should be given to asymptomatic HIV positive children after contact with varicella
D should be given to children receiving inhaled steroid therapy
E is given by intravenous injection

5.7 The following is the current vaccination schedule in England:
A MMR at 12–15 months
B pertussis given at 2, 3, 4 months after estimated date of delivery in preterm infants
C polio and tetanus at school-leaving age
D hepatitis B at delivery
E varicella vaccine at 12 months

5.8 Vaccination against poliomyelitis:
A routinely uses an inactivated oral vaccine
B is contraindicated in preterm neonates
C may result in excretion of the virus for up to 6 weeks
D is contraindicated in children with leukaemia
E must not be administered at the same time as normal immunoglobulin

5.9 The following statements about tuberculin testing are true:
A it may be performed using different strengths of purified protein derivative using the Heaf multiple puncture device
B a Mantoux test result should be observed within 48 hours
C appropriate reactions may be suppressed by infectious mononucleosis
D it should be repeated if the test is negative but an intercurrent respiratory tract infection is present
E it should not be performed within 3 weeks of the administration of a live vaccine

5.10 Influenza vaccination is recommended in children with:
A diabetes mellitus
B cystic fibrosis
C cyanotic heart disease
D nephrotic syndrome receiving alternate day steroids
E chronic renal failure

5.5 A **True**   The Hib vaccine is a conjugated vaccine of purified
     B **False**   capsular polysaccharide with additional protein to aid
     C **False**   immunogenicity. It protects against type b, an
     D **False**   encapsulated variety, which was the major cause of
     E **True**   acute epiglottitis. Three doses are given. As the
                      incidence of such infection decreases after the age of
                      4 years, there is no requirement for a pre-school
                      booster.

5.6 A **False**   Zoster immune globulin (ZIG) has an antibody content
     B **False**   at least 8 times greater than normal immunoglobulin.
     C **False**   It should be given to infants whose mother develops
     D **False**   varicella (not zoster) 1 week before and up to 1 month
     E **False**   after delivery. It should be given to non-immune
                      children receiving high-dose oral steroid therapy. It is
                      an intramuscular injection.

5.7 A **True**   Preterm infants should receive their vaccinations at
     B **False**   the correct times regardless of their prematurity and
     C **True**   not wait until times after their expected date of
     D **False**   delivery. Hepatitis B is not routine but may be given in
     E **False**   specific cases at delivery. Varicella vaccine is not
                      available, routinely, in the UK.

5.8 A **False**   Active oral polio is routinely used in the UK. It may be
     B **False**   excreted for 6 weeks and therefore may pose a risk to
     C **True**   other family members. It may be given to preterm
     D **True**   infants as they leave a neonatal unit but not whilst still
     E **True**   resident. Normal immunoglobulin may negate any
                      immune response.

5.9 A **False**   The Heaf test uses only one strength of PPD. A
     B **False**   Mantoux response is ideally 'read' 48–72 hours after
     C **True**   administration.
     D **True**
     E **True**

5.10 A **True**   These are all recommendations for the use of this
     B **True**   vaccine.
     C **True**
     D **True**
     E **True**

6. Molecular biology

6.1 **In molecular biology:**
  A antibody production may be quantified by Northern blot hybridization
  B RNA is detected by Southern blot hybridization
  C DNA may be cleaved at specific sites by restriction endonucleases
  D exons are transcribed but not translated
  E exons encode gene products

6.2 **Heat shock proteins**
  A only occur in mammals
  B are enzymes
  C are oncogenes
  D are intracytoplasmic receptors
  E may be detected in cells without preceding thermal trauma

6.3 **The polymerase chain reaction**
  A amplifies small amounts of nucleic acid
  B requires a heat sensitive polymerase enzyme
  C quantifies messenger RNA in situ
  D is used in the early diagnosis of HIV infection
  E is based on the ability to produce complementary strands of nucleic acid along a single-stranded denatured DNA template

6.4 **In cell biology:**
  A peroxisomes glycosylate transported proteins
  B membrane bound receptors couple their activation to cellular processes by G proteins
  C alternative splicing may result in two different gene products from the same genetic sequence
  D all DNA resides within the nucleus of the cell
  E active ion transport may be through lipid ion channels

6.1

A	False
B	False
C	True
D	False
E	True

In gene expression, DNA (comprising purine and pyrimidine bases) is transcribed to the primary RNA transcript. The DNA is divided into exons (gene product encoding areas) and introns (variable function including gene regulation). Following the addition of various additional bases, messenger RNA is formed which may then be translated into the gene product. RNA is detected using the Northern blot technique. The Southern blot identifies DNA, and proteins may be detected using the Western blot technique.

6.2

A	False
B	False
C	False
D	False
E	True

Heat shock proteins are highly conserved proteins ubiquitous across the animal world. They are inducible by thermal trauma. Their role in normal cellular function is not fully understood although some may be transcription cofactors involved in gene expression. High levels of some heat shock proteins are detectable in certain autoimmune systemic disorders.

6.3

A	True
B	True
C	False
D	True
E	True

The polymerase chain reaction is a method of producing complementary strands of nucleic acid to a DNA template. This utilizes a heat sensitive DNA polymerase enzyme. Once the strand has been synthesized, the temperature conditions alter and the DNA is denatured. The subsequent denatured single DNA strands then themselves function as the template for the next cycle of DNA synthesis. This technique has been used to identify small amounts of viral nucleic acid, e.g. HIV infection.

6.4

A	False
B	True
C	True
D	False
E	False

Peroxisomes are subcellular organelles which are involved with fatty acid metabolism. Deficiency results in severe metabolic defects. The primary RNA transcript includes exons and transcribed introns which do not code for gene products. The introns are spliced out before the translation of messenger RNA. Differing degrees of splicing result in different gene products. Some DNA exists in the mitochondria and is maternally acquired.

6.5 Proto-oncogenes
  A are only detected in malignant tissue
  B may cause neoplasia by cellular over-expression
  C may be involved in usual cellular function
  D must mutate to cause disease
  E are confined to humans

6.5 A **False** Proto-oncogenes are normal genetic components
B **True** intimately involved in the normal functioning of the
C **True** cell. Over-expression or expression of the gene at an
D **False** incorrect time may result in malignancy by allowing
E **False** disordered cell growth. The proto-oncogene may
mutate itself or be under the erroneous control of a
mutated transcription factor. They are found in other
animals and even in tumorigenic retroviruses.

7. Immunology

7.1 Which of the following statements regarding immunoglobulin classes and function are correct:
  A IgM is a pentamer
  B IgA is always a dimer
  C IgD is a T cell receptor
  D IgG$_4$ is responsible for polysaccharide responses
  E all IgG classes are involved in complement fixation pathways

7.2 Cytokines
  A are steroid receptors
  B include interferons
  C have immunoregulatory functions
  D have growth potentiating effects
  E interact with specific receptors

7.3 Which of the following immune mechanisms are paired correctly with their date of fetal development:
  A thymic development: 14 weeks
  B lymph nodes: 34 weeks
  C splenic development: 8 weeks
  D B cells: 16 weeks
  E Peyer's patches: 20 weeks

7.4 Peanut allergy
  A can be treated with desensitization therapy
  B causes increasingly severe reactions
  C indicates allergy to all nuts
  D may be fatal
  E should be proven using a dietary challenge

7.5 Which of the following neutrophil defects are correctly paired with the resulting clinical disorder:
  A opsonization defect: chronic granulomatous disease
  B motility defect: Chédiak-Higashi disease
  C abnormal morphology: Schwachman syndrome
  D leucocyte membrane adhesion defect: delayed separation of umbilical cord
  E defect in phagocytosis: myeloperoxidase deficiency

7.1 A **True**   All immunoglobulin classes are monomers except IgM
     B **False**   (pentamer) and IgA which may be a dimer when
     C **False**   associated with the secretory component. IgD is a B
     D **False**   cell receptor. IgG_2 is responsible for polysaccharide
     E **False**   responses unlike IgG_4 which is the only subclass not
                       involved in complement fixation.

7.2 A **False**   Cytokines are a group of polypeptides with
     B **True**   immunoregulatory and growth functions.
     C **True**
     D **True**
     E **True**

7.3 A **False**   The following are the correct dates: thymus,
     B **False**   5 weeks; nodes, 8 weeks; and splenic development,
     C **False**   6 weeks.
     D **True**
     E **True**

7.4 A **False**   Peanut allergy is lifelong and is not amenable to
     B **False**   desensitization. Dietary challenge may be potentially
     C **False**   fatal. The severity of future reactions cannot be
     D **True**   predicted on the basis of previous reactions. As
     E **False**   peanuts are legumes rather than tree nuts, there is
                       only about a 10% crossover reaction with nuts such
                       as hazelnuts.

7.5 A **False**   The following are the correct pairings:
     B **False**   opsonization defect: mannan-binding protein
     C **False**   deficiency
     D **True**   killing defect: chronic granulomatous disease and
     E **False**   myeloperoxidase deficiency
                       motility defect: Schwachman syndrome and Job
                       syndrome
                       abnormal morphology: Chédiak-Higashi syndrome.

7.6 Which of the following syndromes are associated with defects of immunity:
  A Turner syndrome
  B Down syndrome
  C Klinefelter syndrome
  D DiGeorge syndrome
  E cri du chat syndrome

7.7 Features of chronic mucocutaneous candidiasis include:
  A preference for candida species other than *C. albicans*
  B male predominance
  C alopecia
  D hyperadrenalism
  E HIV infection

7.8 Recognized features of hypogammaglobulinaemia include:
  A arthritis
  B fungal urinoma
  C *Pneumocystis carinii* pneumonia
  D malabsorption
  E diarrhoea

7.9 Severe combined immunodeficiency (SCID)
  A most commonly affects males
  B presents within the first week of life
  C failure to thrive is uncommon
  D is accompanied by persistent lymphopenia
  E is always accompanied by low immunoglobulin levels at presentation

7.10 Adenosine deaminase deficiency:
  A affects only T cell function
  B presents at the age of 5–10 years
  C is associated with vertebral and costal abnormalities
  D may result in spastic paresis
  E is treated by purine metabolite infusions

7.6 A **True**   Turner syndrome is associated with immunoglobulin
     B **True**   deficiencies. Down syndrome has varied associations
     C **False**   whereas DiGeorge syndrome is accompanied by a
     D **True**   major defect in cellular immunity. The cri du chat
     E **True**   syndrome is associated with defective phagocytosis.

7.7 A **False**   Chronic candidiasis, more commonly seen in girls,
     B **False**   may be associated with a spectrum of autoimmune
     C **True**   disorders including hypoadrenalism and
     D **False**   hypothyroidism. *Candida albicans* predominates
     E **True**   although other species can occur. HIV infection may
                         be complicated by severe and persistent
                         oropharyngeal candidiasis.

7.8 A **True**   Infection, diarrhoea and arthritis are the most
     B **False**   common presentations of hypogammaglobulinaemia.
     C **True**   Whilst T cell deficiencies are more commonly
     D **True**   identified following pneumocystis infection, it can
     E **True**   occur with hypogammaglobulinaemia.

7.9 A **True**   SCID affects males more frequently by 4:1.
     B **False**   Inheritance may be X-linked, sporadic or autosomal
     C **False**   recessive. Presentation occurs within the first few
     D **True**   months with diarrhoea and failure to thrive.
     E **False**   Immunoglobulin levels may initially be normal
                         particularly if there is a high titre of maternally
                         acquired antibody.

7.10 A **False**   Adenosine deaminase deficiency occurs in 15% of
     B **False**   SCID patients. Both cellular and humoral immunity is
     C **True**   affected with clinical presentation within the first few
     D **True**   months of life. 50% of patients display skeletal
     E **False**   abnormalities. Treatment is by bone marrow
                         transplant. The abnormality in purine metabolism may
                         result in CNS defects and paresis.

8. Dermatology

8.1 Which of the following may be associated with a diffuse erythematous maculopapular skin rash:
   A   meningococcus
   B   human herpes type 6 infection
   C   mycoplasma species
   D   measles
   E   *Borrelia burgdorferi*

8.2 Pityriasis rosea:
   A   is usually preceded by a 'herald' patch
   B   is a manifestation of atopy
   C   is aligned along the axis of the ribs
   D   requires steroid therapy
   E   is an autoimmune systemic disorder

8.3 Unilateral limb hypertrophy is associated with:
   A   Klippel-Trenaunay-Weber syndrome
   B   lymphangioma
   C   Sturge-Weber syndrome
   D   dermatomyositis
   E   Gianotti-Crosti syndrome

8.4 Recognized features of the Ehlers-Danlos syndrome include:
   A   cutis hyperelastica
   B   easy bruising
   C   shagreen patch
   D   neonatal hypotonia
   E   tongue fasciculation

8.5 Which of the following may cause hair loss:
   A   telogen effluvium
   B   anorexia nervosa
   C   zinc deficiency
   D   hypoparathyroidism
   E   lead poisoning

8.1
A **True**
B **True**
C **True**
D **True**
E **False**

Whilst classically associated with disseminated purpura, 10–15% of meningococcal septicaemia presents with erythema. This may progress to the more usual situation. HHV6 is accompanied by an erythematous rash, as may measles. Mycoplasma infection may cause many different rashes including typical erythemas.

8.2
A **True**
B **False**
C **True**
D **False**
E **False**

Pityriasis rosea commences with a red/yellow scaly herald patch. This is usually truncal. Similar but smaller lesions occur over the next 2 weeks following the line of the ribs. Usually there is no need for treatment. Resolution occurs in 6 weeks.

8.3
A **True**
B **True**
C **False**
D **False**
E **False**

The Klippel-Trenaunay-Weber syndrome is the association of limb hypertrophy with an underlying vascular malformation. Sturge-Weber is the association of a facial port-wine stain and an angiomatous malformation of the underlying meninges. The Gianotti-Crosti syndrome occurs following a viral illness (often hepatitis B) marked by erythematous papular rash which avoids the trunk.

0.4
A **True**
B **True**
C **False**
D **True**
E **False**

The Ehlers-Danlos syndrome is a heterogenous group of disorders. The majority of sufferers have an autosomal dominant variety. Newborns may have apparent hypotonia. The classic triad includes: extensible skin, connective tissue fragility and joint hypermobility. Shagreen patch is a feature of tuberous sclerosis. Tongue fasciculation occurs in spinal muscular atrophy – another cause of the neonatal 'floppy infant'.

8.5
A **True**
B **True**
C **True**
D **True**
E **False**

Temporary diffuse hair loss due to physical or mental stress (telogen effluvium) occurs. The growing hairs are converted to a resting phase from which they usually recover. Maternal postpartum hair loss is another example. Lead poisoning does not cause hair loss.

8.6 Which of the following are the correct dermatological manifestations of systemic disease:
A perioral lentiginosis: Peutz-Jeghers syndrome
B haemangioma: Kasabach-Merritt syndrome
C symmetrical vesicular rash: dermatitis herpetiformis
D pemphigus: zinc deficiency
E urticaria: Henoch-Schönlein purpura

8.7 Which of the following statements regarding 'nappy rash' are correct:
A perianal candidiasis is the most common cause
B candidiasis may be diagnosed by the absence of satellite lesions
C ammoniacal dermatitis spares the skin creases
D treatment of choice is hydrocortisone cream
E it may be caused by seborrhoeic dermatitis

8.8 Incontinentia pigmenti:
A has a male sex predominance
B is associated with crops of vesicles
C may be associated with seizures
D is associated with a blood basophilia
E is usually apparent in the first week of life

8.9 Erythema neonatorum:
A presents within the first 2 days of life
B is caused by a staphylococcal infection
C causes desquamation
D spares the hands and feet
E is classically an erythematous base containing a papule or apparent pustule

8.10 Pityriasis versicolor:
A is a bacterial infection
B produces erythematous macules
C classically affects the trunk
D is associated with poor hygiene
E is associated with hyperhidrosis

8.6 A **True**   The Kasabach-Merritt syndrome is a consumptive
     B **True**   coagulopathy occurring with platelet sequestration
     C **True**   within a massive haemangioma. Dermatitis
     D **False**   herpetiformis is an itchy symmetrical vesicular rash
     E **True**   on the extensor surfaces. It is associated with auto-
                       immune diseases and coeliac disease. Zinc
                       deficiency is associated with the eczematous
                       acrodermatitis enteropathica. Urticaria may precede
                       the purpura in Henoch-Schönlein purpura.

8.7 A **False**   Nappy rash is usually ammoniacal and usually does
     B **False**   not affect the skin protected by the skin creases.
     C **True**   Candidiasis may secondarily infect this area. Spread
     D **False**   of candida is manifest as satellite lesions. Whilst
     E **True**   hydrocortisone may be occasionally of benefit in
                       severe cases, good hygiene and barrier cream
                       usually suffice with antifungal medication as
                       necessary.

8.8 A **False**   This rare condition affects females. The crops of
     B **True**   vesicles appear in the first 2 weeks of life followed by
     C **True**   warty papules and finally pigmentary changes. Dental
     D **False**   and ocular anomalies may occur together with
     E **True**   seizures. Mental retardation occurs rarely. An
                       eosinophilia commonly accompanies this diagnosis.

8.9 A **True**   This is very common and may be florid. The central
     B **False**   papule contains eosinophils but this is not allergic in
     C **False**   nature.
     D **False**
     E **True**

8.10 A **False**   The fungus, *Malassezia furfur*, is the responsible
     B **False**   agent in truncal regions of poor hygiene and
     C **True**   excessive sweating. It is a scaly, light brown eruption.
     D **True**   Antifungals remain the mainstay of therapy.
     E **True**

9. Child abuse

9.1 Which of the following features on skull radiography would be suggestive of non-accidental injury:
- A parietal bone fracture
- B occipital bone fracture
- C fracture width exceeding 3 mm
- D a fracture crossing suture lines
- E a 'growing' fracture

9.2 The following statements regarding child abuse are correct:
- A first born children are more likely to suffer abuse
- B children over 4 years of age are more at risk of severe abuse
- C sexual abuse is more commonly perpetrated by men
- D abuse is suspected in 10% of the UK population under the age of 12 years
- E there is no relation to whether the parent was abused as a child

9.3 Fractures suggestive of child abuse include:
- A rib fractures
- B clavicular fractures
- C scapular fractures
- D metaphyseal fractures
- E fractures at differing ages of resolution

9.4 Clinical features which may indicate sexual abuse include:
- A soft palatal petechiae
- B positive reflex anal dilatation in the presence of constipation
- C adhesions of labia minora
- D perianal candidosis
- E perianal abscess

9.1	A	**False**	Head injury is a common manifestation of abuse and the major cause of mortality. 40–70% of physically abused children suffer some degree of head injury. Single linear narrow parietal fractures affecting one bone have a low specificity for abuse. The occipital bone is so thick that a considerable force is necessary to cause a fracture, hence a high level of suspicion is mandatory. A wide fracture or a 'growing' fracture which is indicative of a dural tear and underlying brain injury are highly suspicious of non-accidental injury. 'Growing' fractures only occur in infancy.
	B	**True**	
	C	**True**	
	D	**True**	
	E	**True**	

9.2	A	**True**	First born children are seemingly more at risk as are children below 2 years. Abuse is believed to be suspected in 4% of children below the age of 12 years. If a parent was abused, his/her children are statistically 20 times more at risk than the general paediatric population.
	B	**False**	
	C	**True**	
	D	**False**	
	E	**False**	

9.3	A	**True**	No fracture is pathognomonic of child abuse. Clavicular fractures are common innocent fractures and may occur at the time of delivery. Metaphyseal and epiphyseal injuries are classic fractures associated with abuse. They occur as a result of acceleration/deceleration injuries, e.g. shaking. Rib fractures are often occult and occur as a result of direct violence.
	B	**False**	
	C	**True**	
	D	**True**	
	E	**True**	

9.4	A	**True**	Signs of sexual abuse are varied and rarely specific. A positive reflex anal dilatation test often occurs in cases of long-standing constipation as well as chronic anal penetration. Soft palate petechiae may indicate infectious mononucleosis but also forced oral penetration. Labial adhesions may be developmental in origin but also represent the results of physical trauma. Perianal abscesses may be a feature of Crohn's disease.
	B	**False**	
	C	**True**	
	D	**False**	
	E	**False**	

9.5 Which of the following are useful time approximations when ageing an injury considered to be non-accidental:
  A brown bruise: less than 24 hours since injury
  B slower resolution with bruises of the pinna
  C periosteal formation: 4–5 days
  D callus formation: more than 14 days
  E yellowing of bruise: greater than 72 hours

9.6 Which of the following features of burns may be suggestive of non-accidental injury:
  A scalds affecting the upper trunk
  B 'hole in the doughnut' buttock burn
  C symmetrical lower limb scald
  D round burns with central necrosis
  E child with scald exhibiting 'frozen watchfulness'

9.5 A **False** Ageing of bruises is variable. Avascular areas may
B **True** evolve at a slower rate. One rough guide is:
C **False** • less than 24 hours: red/purple
D **True** • 12–48 hours: purple/blue
E **True** • 48–72 hours: brown
• greater than 72 hours: yellow
Dating of fractures is of medicolegal significance. The following remains a rough guide:
• resolution of soft tissue swelling: 4–10 days
• periosteal formation: 10–14 days
• loss fracture line definition: 14–21 days
• callus: 14–45 days

9.6 A **False** All burns and scalds need a careful examination and
B **True** explanation. Some are more likely to be associated
C **True** with child abuse. Some burns may indicate the
D **True** implement used, e.g. poker. The shape of the lesion
E **True** may indicate the nature of the problem. Scalds from accidentally tipping hot fluid over the child are usually uneven and affect the upper trunk. Forceful placing of the buttocks on a hot surface produces a burn with central perianal sparing – the 'hole in the doughnut' sign. Round burns with central necrosis suggest cigarette burns. However, the whole child should be considered including an awareness of the silent 'frozen watchfulness' demeanour.

10. Haematology and oncology

10.1 A peripheral blood eosinophilia is a recognized feature of:
  A   Hodgkin's lymphoma
  B   Wiskott-Aldrich syndrome
  C   Schwachman syndrome
  D   iron deficiency anaemia
  E   ataxia-telangiectasia

10.2 Which of the following statements regarding neuroblastoma are correct:
  A   neuroblastoma is the most common extracranial solid tumour in childhood
  B   metastatic disease always confers a poor prognosis
  C   infants less than 1 year of age have the worst prognosis
  D   20% arise in the adrenal cortex
  E   thoracic neuroblastoma carries the worst prognosis

10.3 In homozygous sickle cell disease:
  A   aplastic crises are precipitated by cytomegalovirus infection
  B   dactylitis is often the initial vaso-occlusive crisis
  C   elevated HbF levels are associated with increased risk of painful crises
  D   diagnosis cannot be made in the neonatal period
  E   nocturnal enuresis is more common than in the general population

10.4 Poor prognostic features of survival in acute lymphoblastic leukaemia include:
  A   male sex
  B   age above 5 years
  C   peripheral white cell count exceeding 20×10^9/l
  D   thrombocytopenia
  E   Hb less than 8.0 g/dl

10.1 A **True**   Eosinophil counts vary with age (reduced during the
      B **True**   neonatal period) and a diurnal variation with evening
      C **False**   accentuation. The major causes include: allergy/
      D **False**   atopy; parasitic disease; drugs including antibiotics;
      E **False**   haematological (Hodgkin's lymphoma, CML);
                    autoimmune disorders; chronic infections; and
                    disseminated malignancy. The Wiskott-Aldrich
                    syndrome, an immunodeficiency, is an X-linked
                    disease featuring chronic thrombocytopenia,
                    eczema and recurrent infections. Schwachman
                    syndrome comprises metaphyseal chondroplasia,
                    short stature, neutropenia and exocrine pancreatic
                    insufficiency. The sweat test is normal but the serum
                    immunoreactive trypsin level is low.

10.2 A **True**   Neuroblastoma is a common paediatric malignancy.
      B **False**   The median incidence is 2 years and presentation
      C **False**   after 7 years is uncommon. Prognosis in the under-
      D **False**   1-years is good as some show spontaneous tumour
      E **False**   regression. 60% arise in the abdomen. Half of these
                    occur in the adrenal medulla. Thoracic primaries are
                    often localized and discovered incidentally. These
                    are often relatively well-differentiated and therefore
                    have a better prognosis. In infants less than 1 year
                    widespread metastases to skin, liver or bone marrow
                    occur with a good prognosis due to spontaneous
                    regression.

10.3 A **False**   Aplastic crises are usually a feature of parvovirus
      B **True**   B19 infection. Vaso-occlusive crises affect active
      C **False**   bone marrow and in infants this includes the marrow
      D **False**   of the metacarpals. Dactylitis is one of the common
      E **True**   presentations. Elevated HbF levels are protective
                    against vaso-occlusive crises. Neonatal diagnosis
                    may be made both by sensitive haemoglobin
                    electrophoresis and molecular biological methods.
                    Repeated renal infarcts result in loss of renal
                    concentrating power leading to nocturnal enuresis.

10.4 A **True**   Various factors have been utilized to provide
      B **False**   prognostic indicators. These include: sex, age
      C **True**   (worse prognosis if under 1 or above 8 years), race,
      D **False**   immunological type, blast count (white count above
      E **False** 20–50×10^9/l), chromosomal markers and CNS
                    involvement.

10.5 **Which of the following are causes of a macrocytosis:**
A Imerslund-Gräsbeck syndrome
B reticulocytosis
C hypothyroidism
D sideroblastic anaemia
E lead toxicity

10.6 **Recognized causes of purpura include:**
A Kawasaki's disease
B post-splenectomy
C Coxsackie infection
D scurvy
E TAR syndrome

10.7 **Which of the following coagulation factors are tested using the prothrombin time:**
A factor II
B factor VII
C factor X
D factor V
E protein C

10.8 **Which of the following coagulation deficiencies are likely in a child with an abnormal partial thromboplastin time, normal thrombin time and normal prothrombin time:**
A disseminated intravascular coagulation
B heparin effect
C thrombocytopenia
D Glanzmann's disease
E haemophilia B

10.9 **The following statements regarding acute idiopathic thrombocytopenic purpura are correct:**
A marked splenomegaly is common
B bleeding is usually intra-articular
C the aetiology is often postviral
D treatment with immunoglobulin is curative
E may be the presenting feature of systemic lupus erythematosus

10.5 A **True**   Macrocytosis is normal in preterm infants. Other
      B **True**   causes include: vitamin B_{12} and folate deficiency,
      C **True**   liver disease, hypothyroidism, aplastic anaemia and
      D **False**   reticulocytosis. The Imerslund-Gräsbeck syndrome
      E **False**   results in B_{12} deficiency by a failure of uptake of the
                       B_{12}-intrinsic factor complex by the ileum.
                       Microcytosis is a feature of sideroblastic anaemia.

10.6 A **True**   Purpura occurs usually in the presence of low or
      B **True**   normal platelets. It may occur in the presence of
      C **True**   thrombocytosis with haemorrhagic tendency
      D **True**   including after splenectomy. Kawasaki's disease is a
      E **True**   vasculitis which may occasionally result in purpura.
                       Thrombocytopenia, due to coxsackie infection, may
                       occur. The TAR syndrome is the association of
                       thrombocytopenia with absent radii.

10.7 A **True**   The prothrombin time is an indicator of the extrinsic
      B **True**   coagulation mechanism. Abnormalities may be due
      C **True**   to deficiencies of: prothrombin (factor II), factors V,
      D **True**   VII, X and fibrinogen.
      E **False**

10.8 A **False**   This combination of coagulation deficiencies may
      B **False**   result from deficiencies of: factors VIII, IX, XI and
      C **False**   XII. Deficiency of factor IX results in Christmas
      D **False**   disease (haemophilia B).
      E **True**

10.9 A **False**   Acute ITP is common and usually follows a viral
      B **False**   illness. Occasionally it may be mistaken for the
      C **True**   presentation of SLE particularly in teenage girls who
      D **False**   are less likely to develop classic acute ITP. Bleeding
      E **True**   is often mucosal or beneath the skin. Marked
                       splenomegaly is rare although the spleen may be
                       slightly palpable. Usually no treatment is necessary
                       but in severe cases symptomatic therapy with an
                       elevation in platelet count may be produced using
                       intravenous γ-globulin infusions.

10.10 Haemorrhagic disease of the newborn:
  A is reliably prevented by a single dose of oral vitamin K
  B never occurs after 5 days of age
  C may cause severe intracranial haemorrhage
  D may be the presenting feature of neonatal hepatitis
  E is more common in bottle-fed than breast-fed babies

10.11 Hepatoblastoma:
  A has an age predominance below 3 years of age
  B is associated with infants of diabetic mothers
  C usually presents with jaundice
  D has a female sex predominance
  E is often associated with an elevated serum α-fetoprotein level

10.12 The following are common presentations of acute lymphoblastic leukaemia:
  A spinal pain
  B painful limp
  C fever
  D seizure
  E hepatosplenomegaly

10.13 Features of craniopharyngioma and its treatment include:
  A presentation with evidence of raised intracranial pressure
  B it comprises 20% of paediatric intracranial tumours
  C it causes visual field defects
  D hyponatraemia is frequent
  E chemotherapy is the treatment of choice

10.14 Complications of iron overload include:
  A pubertal delay
  B cardiomyopathy
  C hypothyroidism
  D tetany
  E deafness

10.10 A **False**   Neonatal haemorrhagic disease is reliably prevented
       B **False**   by intramuscular administration of vitamin K but not
       C **True**   by oral administration. This is exacerbated in breast-
       D **True**   fed babies or those with unsuspected malabsorption
       E **False**   or liver disease. Late onset haemorrhage may occur
                        after 2 weeks and usually presents as severe
                        intracranial haemorrhage. Breast-fed babies who do
                        not receive parenteral vitamin K should receive
                        several oral doses for protection.

10.11 A **True**   75% of cases present before the age of 3 years.
       B **False**   Males are twice as commonly affected as females.
       C **False**   Abdominal distension is the most common
       D **False**   presentation. Infants with Beckwith syndrome are at
       E **True**   risk of hepatoblastoma unlike infants of diabetic
                        mothers. Other associations include: Sotos
                        syndrome, Wilson's disease, tyrosinaemia, glycogen
                        storage disorders and fetal alcohol syndrome.

10.12 A **True**   All may present in many ways including features of
       B **True**   marrow failure, e.g. bleeding, fever and infection.
       C **True**   Pathological fractures may occur as may non-
       D **False**   specific bone pain. CNS involvement rarely results in
       E **True**   a presentation of seizures.

10.13 A **True**   Craniopharyngioma usually presents with evidence
       B **False**   of raised intracranial pressure. Visual field defects
       C **True**   are common. They account for 6–13% of intracranial
       D **False**   tumours. Vasopressin deficiency may occur leading
       E **False**   to hypernatraemia. Hormonal supplementation is
                        often necessary. Surgery is the treatment of choice.

10.14 A **True**   Problems of iron overload may complicate
       B **True**   thalassaemia despite the use of chelation therapy.
       C **True**   Cardiac complications include cardiomyopathy and
       D **True**   myocardial dysfunction. Growth retardation is
       E **False**   common and may be due to several different factors
                        including: hypothyroidism, hypoparathyroidism,
                        growth hormone deficiency and IGF-1 deficiency
                        due to liver dysfunction. Pubertal delay and
                        hypogonadism occurs. However chelation therapy
                        with desferrioxamine may be complicated by bloody
                        diarrhoea, infection, hypersensitivity, growth failure,
                        ophthalmic problems and ototoxicity.

10.15 Which of the following statements relating to β-thalassaemia major is correct:
   A it arises from excessive synthesis of defective β-haemoglobin chains
   B inheritance is autosomal dominant with variable penetrance
   C it confers relative protection from falciparum malaria
   D elevation of HbA_2 level occurs
   E is associated with Yersinia enteritis

10.16 Features of iron deficiency anaemia include:
   A elevated serum ferritin
   B reticulocytosis
   C growth retardation
   D cognitive impairment
   E encephalopathy

10.17 Thrombocytosis occurs in:
   A chronic gastrointestinal haemorrhage
   B Kawasaki's disease
   C haemolytic-uraemic syndrome
   D systemic lupus erythematosus
   E iron deficiency anaemia

10.18 Nephroblastoma:
   A usually presents with haematuria
   B is associated with Beckwith syndrome
   C metastasizes to the liver
   D is radiosensitive
   E is often calcified on plain abdominal X-ray

10.15   A **False**   Homozygous β-thalassaemia is a common inherited
        B **False**   condition resulting from defective β-globin
        C **True**   production. Inheritance is autosomal recessive. The
        D **True**   deletions occur on chromosome 11. The deletion
        E **True**   may confer some resistance to falciparum malaria –
                       hence the geographical distribution. Early
                       erythrocyte death results in severe and progressive
                       anaemia necessitating regular blood transfusions.
                       Hb electrophoresis shows reduced HbA, increased
                       HbA$_2$ and the presence of fetal haemoglobin.
                       Yersinia enteritis occurs as a complication of
                       chelation therapy.

10.16   A **False**   Serum ferritin represents the level of iron stores
        B **False**   although it may be elevated in inflammatory
        C **True**   conditions. Free erythrocyte protoporphyrin levels
        D **True**   are elevated. Haemolysis or extreme anaemia may
        E **False**   be associated with reticulocytosis but not usually in
                       simple iron deficiency. Growth retardation and
                       cognitive impairment are non-haematological effects
                       of iron deficiency. Encephalopathy is a feature of
                       lead toxicity.

10.17   A **True**   Elevated platelet counts are present in vasculitic
        B **True**   disorders or in the presence of gastrointestinal blood
        C **False**   loss. Additional causes include: post-splenectomy,
        D **False**   malignancy, myeloproliferative disorders and iron
        E **True**   deficiency. Thrombocytopenia occurs with SLE and
                       the haemolytic-uraemic syndrome.

10.18   A **False**   The majority of Wilm's tumours (nephroblastoma)
        B **True**   present with an abdominal mass. Haematuria
        C **True**   occurs in 20–30% of cases. Some cases are
        D **True**   associated with Beckwith syndrome. Metastasis is
        E **False**   primarily to the lungs, regional nodes and the liver.
                       Treatment uses various modalities but these
                       tumours are generally radiosensitive. Radiological
                       calcification is, characteristically, more of a feature
                       of a neuroblastoma.

10.19 Von Willebrand's disease:
- A is associated with mucosal surface bleeding
- B is associated with an abnormal Hess test
- C is associated with a platelet aggregation defect to ristocetin
- D is autosomal recessive
- E is treated with cryoprecipitate

10.20 Haemophagocytic histiocytosis:
- A may be associated with Epstein-Barr virus infection
- B is highly chemotherapy sensitive
- C may be diagnosed on bone marrow biopsy
- D may be familial
- E causes hepatomegaly

10.19　A　**True**　　Von Willebrand's disease is the commonest
　　　　B　**True**　　congenital bleeding disorder. Whilst failure of
　　　　C　**True**　　platelet aggregation to ristocetin is a feature,
　　　　D　**False**　 diagnosis rests on the demonstration of abnormal
　　　　E　**True**　　levels of Von Willebrand's factor and other factor VIII components. Mucosal bleeding, particularly after dental extraction, is more common than haemoarthroses as in haemophilia A. Inheritance is autosomal dominant. Treatment is usually by fresh frozen plasma infusion although cryoprecipitate administration may be used. Prolonged bleeding time and abnormal Hess test occur.

10.20　A　**True**　　The histiocytoses are a heterogenous group of
　　　　B　**False**　 disorders. Diagnosis and treatment are often difficult
　　　　C　**True**　　and often chemotherapy is of little benefit. Acquired
　　　　D　**True**　　forms may be associated with glandular fever.
　　　　E　**True**　　Diagnosis depends upon the demonstration of haemophagocytosis in bone marrow, liver or CSF. There are familial varieties.

11. Metabolism

11.1 Gaucher's disease:
 A may cause coxalgia
 B is invariably associated with splenomegaly
 C is caused by a deficiency of glucocerebrosidase
 D results in elevation of serum angiotensin converting enzyme
 E is untreatable

11.2 Which of the following may be used in an emergency to treat a serum potassium level of 8.9 mmol/l:
 A salbutamol
 B calcium gluconate
 C oral phosphate
 D glucose-insulin combination
 E magnesium salt

11.3 Galactosaemia:
 A may present with septicaemia
 B is confirmed by a positive urinary reducing substance assay in over 80% of cases
 C will only cause cataracts after several months of age
 D is a cause of an unconjugated hyperbilirubinaemia
 E cannot be biochemically diagnosed on enzyme assay after a recent blood transfusion

11.1 A **True**   Gaucher's disease is an autosomal recessive
      B **False**   disorder caused by a deficiency of glucocerebro-
      C **True**   sidase. This results in an accumulation of the
      D **True**   glycolipid, glucocerebroside, in the
      E **False**   reticuloendothelial system. Whilst the prevalence is
                       higher in various Jewish groups, the incidence in
                       non-Jewish groups approximates to 1:100 000.
                       There are several types conforming to the various
                       genotypic mutations. Non-neurological
                       manifestations include hepatosplenomegaly and
                       skeletal disease. The former is not invariable.
                       Skeletal problems include coxalgia, pathological
                       fractures and infarction. Marrow replacement
                       manifests as haematological disturbances. Elevated
                       SACE levels occur due to activation of the
                       macrophages. Diagnosis is by measurement of
                       leucocyte glucocerebrosidase or direct gene
                       analysis. Treatment is based on supportive therapy
                       and the use of intravenous mannose-terminated
                       glucocerebrosidase of human placental origin.

11.2 A **True**   The most common cause of acute hyperkalaemia is
      B **True**   renal failure. In the presence of an arrhythmia,
      C **False**   intravenous calcium is the treatment of choice. If
      D **True**   there is no evidence of life-threatening arrhythmia,
      E **False**   nebulized or intravenous β_2-agonist will cause a
                       rapid fall in serum potassium. Other therapies
                       include: calcium resonium. Oral phosphate is
                       ineffective in the acute situation. Magnesium salts
                       are used as muscle relaxants.

11.3 A **True**   Galactosaemia presents as a Gram-negative
      B **False**   septicaemia in one-third of cases. There is often
      C **False**   associated liver and haematological disturbances.
      D **True**   The presence of urinary reducing substances is a
      E **True**   screen but not confirmatory and sufferers may
                       occasionally be missed when the urine is normal.
                       Diagnosis is by enzyme assay in erythrocytes
                       (galactose-1-phosphate uridyl transferase). This is
                       unreliable following a recent transfusion. Cataracts
                       may occur early in the disease shortly after birth.
                       Initially there may be an unconjugated
                       hyperbilirubinaemia although this is replaced by a
                       conjugated variety when significant liver impairment
                       has occurred.

11.4 Which of the following may be a cause of hyponatraemia:
- A Legionnaire's disease
- B Bartter syndrome
- C cystic fibrosis
- D urinary tract infection
- E distal renal tubular acidosis

11.5 Maple syrup urine disease:
- A is an organic aciduria
- B is associated with elevated plasma levels of leucine, isoleucine and valine
- C presents with jaundice and liver failure
- D is a cause of neonatal encephalopathy
- E causes neonatal hiccoughs

11.6 Which of the following statements regarding neonatal metabolic disorders is true:
- A all cause acidosis
- B all present with hypoglycaemia
- C they usually present at or immediately after delivery
- D they often demonstrate an enlarged anion gap
- E heavy ketonuria is rare

11.4
A	**True**
B	**True**
C	**True**
D	**True**
E	**False**

Hyponatraemia may arise from several disturbances. Salt depletion through a combination of excess loss (sweat or urine) accounts for the disordered sodium level in cystic fibrosis (pseudo-Bartter syndrome) and urinary tract infection (particularly if there is an element of renal obstruction). Inappropriate vasopressin secretion often accompanies respiratory infections of many varieties including atypical pneumonias and bronchiolitis. Bartter syndrome is probably due to abnormal function of the renal juxtaglomerular organs. Clinically, the child may fail to thrive with anorexia, polydipsia and polyuria. Biochemically the electrolyte profile manifests hypokalaemia alkalosis with hyponatraemia. Distal renal tubular acidosis causes acidosis, hyperchloraemia, normal anion gap and normonatraemia.

11.5
A	**False**
B	**True**
C	**False**
D	**True**
E	**False**

Maple syrup urine disease is an aminoaciduria with elevated plasma and urine levels of valine, leucine and isoleucine. This condition usually presents with neurological deterioration into apnoea and coma with seizures. Liver failure is not a presenting feature. Neonatal hiccoughs are not common. They may be noted in those suffering non-ketotic hyperglycinaemia.

11.6
A	**False**
B	**False**
C	**False**
D	**True**
E	**False**

Whilst many metabolic disorders cause hypoglycaemia and acidosis, many do not. Non-ketotic hyperglycinaemia does not cause either but results in marked neurological deterioration. Tyrosinaemia usually causes liver dysfunction but little acidosis or hypoglycaemia. Many disorders do not appear immediately as they require an accumulation of toxic metabolites which have previously been detoxified by the placenta. Many disorders produce an enlarged anion gap. Heavy ketonuria is rare in the neonatal period but its presence is strongly suggestive of an organic aciduric disorder.

11.7 Recognized features of peroxisomal disorders include:
 A hypertonia
 B early seizures
 C pigmentary retinopathy
 D small fontanelle
 E renal cysts

11.8 Causes of neonatal hypoglycaemia include:
 A nesidioblastosis
 B William's syndrome
 C intrauterine growth retardation
 D polycythaemia
 E neonatal diabetes mellitus

11.9 Which of the following statements regarding hypothermia are correct:
 A thermogenesis fails when the core temperature falls below 32°C
 B resuscitation of children must not be discontinued until the core temperature is above 32°C
 C pupillary reaction decreases with increasing hypothermia
 D cardiac defibrillation is not affected by core temperature
 E hypoglycaemia is a frequent concomitant of hypothermia

11.10 Urea cycle defects:
 A cause hypoglycaemia
 B are treated by regular haemodialysis
 C may be suspected in the presence of hyperammonaemia
 D may be associated with a respiratory alkalosis
 E cause characteristic amino acid profile

11.7

A	False	Peroxisomes are subcellular organelles.
B	True	Abnormalities result in dysmorphic individuals with
C	True	profound hypotonia. Large fontanelles occur.
D	False	Zellweger syndrome remains the best-known
E	True	condition. Additional features include renal cysts, mental retardation and pigmentary retinopathy. Biochemically, peroxisomal disorders are associated with fatty acid metabolism.

11.8

A	True	Recent studies suggest that cerebral electrical
B	False	activity is affected when the blood glucose level
C	True	decreases below 2.6 mmol/l. Preterm infants are
D	True	often affected as are intrauterine growth retarded
E	False	infants who may have insufficient glycogen stores. Hyperinsulinism (infants of diabetic mothers; nesidioblastosis; Beckwith syndrome, severe haemolytic disease and islet cell adenoma) is another cause. Others include sepsis, hypoxia, cold stress and polycythaemia. William's syndrome causes hypercalcaemia and neonatal diabetes mellitus causes hyperglycaemia.

11.9

A	True	Accidental hypothermia often accompanies
B	True	accidents such as drowning. Neurological function is
C	True	affected by hypothermia with fixed pupils occurring.
D	False	However, resuscitation must not be discontinued
E	True	until rewarming has occurred as the prognosis may not be as dismal as expected with full recovery in many documented cases. Thermogenesis fails below 32°C, therefore, active rewarming is necessary in addition to supportive passive warming. Defibrillation may be ineffective in the presence of severe hypothermia.

11.10

A	False	Urea cycle defects are rare. They may present in the
B	False	neonatal period. Biochemical features include:
C	True	alkalosis, hyperammonaemia and typical amino acid
D	True	profiles depending upon which defect occurs. Some
E	True	varieties cause neurological and hepatic dysfunction which may mimic Reye syndrome. Haemodialysis may be of benefit acutely but regular therapy is dietary and detoxification using sodium benzoate and phenylacetate.

11.11 Which of the following are appropriate metabolic responses to acute stress:
   A increased secretion of insulin
   B increased lipolysis
   C increased secretion of vasopressin
   D decreased gluconeogenesis
   E increased growth hormone secretion

11.12 Recognized causes of hypocalcaemia include:
   A hyperparathyroidism
   B hypervitaminosis D
   C sarcoidosis
   D medullary carcinoma of the thyroid
   E Addison's disease

11.13 Features of glycogen storage disorders include:
   A short stature
   B neutropenia
   C rickets
   D hepatomegaly
   E hepatoblastoma

11.14 Hepatomegaly is a recognized feature of:
   A tyrosinaemia
   B Crigler-Najjar syndrome
   C non-ketotic hyperglycinaemia
   D isovaleric acidaemia
   E glycogen storage disease type II

11.15 Which of the following would suggest a diagnosis of medium chain acyl coenzyme A dehydrogenase deficiency (MCAD):
   A sudden infant death
   B heavy ketonuria
   C hypoglycaemia
   D hyperinsulinaemia
   E hyperfattyacidaemia

11.11	A	**False**	The metabolic response to stress activates and modulates the following increased hormone secretion: adrenaline, cortisol, glucagon and growth hormone. Insulin secretion is inhibited. Lipolysis and gluconeogenesis are other mechanisms for increasing plasma glucose levels which occur during stress.
	B	**True**	
	C	**True**	
	D	**False**	
	E	**True**	

11.12	A	**False**	All are causes of hypercalcaemia except medullary thyroid cancer. In this situation there may be chronic excess secretion of biologically active calcitonin. Whilst calcitonin should decrease the serum calcium level, clinically hypocalcaemia does not occur.
	B	**False**	
	C	**False**	
	D	**False**	
	E	**False**	

11.13	A	**True**	Glycogen storage disorders are a heterogenous group of disorders with differing clinical features and prognoses. Severe hypoglycaemia, hepatomegaly and growth failure are features of the most common type I disease. Neutropenia is an accompanying feature of type Ib. Hepatic adenomata may occur in older children and adolescents with type I. Type II is usually fatal.
	B	**True**	
	C	**False**	
	D	**True**	
	E	**True**	

11.14	A	**True**	The Crigler-Najjar syndrome includes two defects of bilirubin metabolism. Both cause marked unconjugated hyperbilirubinaemia requiring phototherapy. Isovaleric acidaemia is an organic acidaemia with the accompanying classic odour of 'sweaty feet'.
	B	**False**	
	C	**False**	
	D	**False**	
	E	**True**	

11.15	A	**True**	A proportion of 'sudden infant death/cot death' babies are believed to have this defect of fat β-oxidation. In this situation the infant is unable to metabolize mobilized fatty acids. Therefore there is hypoglycaemia, hyperfattyacidaemia with hypoketonaemia. Hypoinsulinism occurs. MCAD is the most common type of this family of disorders. Other presentations include Reye syndrome-like illness and cardiomyopathy. Treatment is avoidance of starvation particularly during periods of stress including times of illness.
	B	**False**	
	C	**True**	
	D	**False**	
	E	**True**	

12. Neurology

12.1 **Recognized causes of acute ataxia include:**
- A occult neuroblastoma
- B paracetamol overdose
- C varicella infection
- D maple syrup urine disease
- E Refsum's disease

12.2 **In cases of salt water drowning:**
- A fixed dilated pupils always indicates irreversible brain death
- B pupils are usually pin-point
- C hypernatraemia is a constant feature
- D acute demyelination occurs
- E cerebral oedema is rare

12.3 **Which of the following are indications for intubation of a child following a head injury:**
- A modified Glasgow Coma Score of 11
- B unilateral fixed dilated pupil
- C absent gag reflex
- D seizure
- E decorticate posturing

12.4 **Recognized causes of macrocephaly include:**
- A Seckel syndrome
- B neurofibromatosis type 1
- C congenital cytomegalovirus infection
- D Rett syndrome
- E communicating hydrocephalus

12.1 A **True**   Acute ataxia is relatively common. Poisoning,
      B **False**   accidental or intentional, is common particularly with
      C **True**   anticonvulsants or alcohol. Acute ataxia following
      D **True**   viral illnesses may represent encephalopathy due to
      E **False**   direct infection or, more commonly, parainfectious
                       phenomenon. Other aetiologies include occult
                       neuroblastoma; metabolic diseases including
                       aminoacidurias; hypothyroidism; posterior fossa
                       haemorrhage and the Guillain-Barré syndrome.
                       Refsum's disease, due to a deficiency of phytanic
                       acid oxidase, causes chronic progressive ataxia.

12.2 A **False**   Salt water drowning is often accompanied by
      B **False**   hypothermia. Pupillary changes are unreliable
      C **False**   indicators of cerebral function in the presence of a
      D **False**   hypothermic core temperature. Resuscitation should
      E **True**   not be abandoned until rewarming has occurred.
                       Hypernatraemia may occur but is not a constant
                       feature. Acute demyelination usually follows rapid
                       correction of profound hyponatraemia. Cerebral
                       oedema may accompany resuscitation of a hypoxic
                       insult but is more a feature of fresh water drowning.

12.3 A **False**   Absolute indications for intubation following head
      B **True**   injury include: inadequate respiration; absent gag
      C **True**   reflex; depression of the modified Glasgow Coma
      D **False**   Score of 8 or less; and signs of brain herniation
      E **True**   including unilateral pupillary dilatation. Decorticate
                       posturing indicates marked intracranial injury and is
                       another indication for intubation.

12.4 A **False**   Macrocephaly is most commonly familial. Acquired
      B **True**   causes include subdural collections and
      C **False**   hydrocephalus. Other causes include diseases
      D **False**   characterized by increased brain mass, e.g. Tay-
      E **True**   Sachs disease. 45% of those with neurofibromatosis
                       have relative macrocephaly. Seckel and Rett
                       syndromes are causes of microcephaly and this is
                       also a feature of some congenital infections.

12.5 Which of the following pupillary signs are correctly linked to the corresponding pathophysiology:
    A fixed pin-point pupils: midbrain lesion
    B fixed mid-size pupils: barbiturate poisoning
    C unilateral dilated pupil: tentorial herniation
    D fixed dilated pupils: hyperthermia
    E small reactive pupils: pontine lesion

12.6 Recognized features of tuberous sclerosis include:
    A café-au-lait patches
    B axillary freckling
    C adenoma sebaceum
    D gyral calcification
    E ungual fibromata

12.7 Features of a headache suspicious of underlying intracranial pathology include:
    A evening exacerbation
    B crushing sensation
    C scalp tenderness
    D absence of relief from simple analgesia
    E photophobia

12.8 Features of a meningomyelocele suggestive of a poor prognosis include:
    A hydrocephalus after surgery
    B thoracic lesion
    C associated visceral abnormalities
    D associated hemivertebrae
    E neuropathic bladder

12.9 Febrile convulsions
    A occur in 15% of the population
    B may occur in the neonatal period
    C may be prevented using phenytoin
    D may be familial
    E recur in about 3% of children

12.5	A	**False**	The correct pairings are:
	B	**False**	fixed pin-point pupils: metabolic disorders; opiate/
	C	**True**	barbiturates
	D	**False**	fixed mid-size pupils: midbrain lesion
	E	**False**	fixed dilated pupils: hypothermia; severe hypoxia; post-seizure; barbiturate poisoning (late sign); irreversible brain damage
			small reactive pupils: metabolic disorders; medullary lesion

12.6	A	**False**	Tuberous sclerosis is a neurocutaneous syndrome
	B	**False**	characterized by facial angiofibromata (adenoma
	C	**True**	sebaceum), seizures and mental retardation. Other
	D	**False**	features include periventricular cranial tubers,
	E	**True**	cardiac and renal tumours and characteristic skin stigmata. Café-au-lait patches and axillary freckling are features of neurofibromatosis type 1. Gyral calcification occurs in another neurocutaneous syndrome, the Sturge-Weber syndrome.

12.7	A	**False**	There are no pathognomonic features for intracranial
	B	**False**	pathology. Suspicious symptoms suggestive of an
	C	**False**	intracranial tumour include: early morning headache;
	D	**True**	pain waking at night; lack of relief from analgesia;
	E	**False**	exacerbation when coughing and additional neurological signs such as head tilt.

12.8	A	**False**	Poor prognostic indicators associated with
	B	**True**	meningomyelocele are: thoracolumbar lesions;
	C	**True**	severe paraplegia below a level of L3; kyphosis;
	D	**False**	hydrocephalus before surgical closure; intracranial
	E	**True**	birth injury; and severe congenital deformities. The majority of infants will develop hydrocephalus after closure of the lesion.

12.9	A	**False**	Febrile convulsions occur in 2–3% of children
	B	**False**	between the ages of 6 months and 6 years. One-
	C	**False**	third have a family history. Approximately one-third
	D	**True**	will suffer further febrile seizures. Prophylaxis with
	E	**False**	phenobarbitone, phenytoin and valproate does not seem to be successful.

12.10 Absence seizures:
   A may occur in the absence of supportive EEG data
   B are rare in the prepubertal age group
   C may progress to generalized seizures
   D are best treated with vigabatrin
   E usually have an underlying cortical focal lesion

12.11 Infantile spasms:
   A indicate underlying brain disorder
   B are incompatible with normal development
   C respond to valproate
   D are usually associated with electrolyte abnormalities
   E are usually indicated by hypsarrhythmia on the EEG

12.12 Which of the following are consistent with the diagnosis of 'brain death':
   A absent corneal reflex in an infant of 27 weeks' gestation
   B fixed dilated pupils with a core temperature of 31°C
   C absent cough reflex whilst receiving phenobarbitone
   D absent doll's eyes manoeuvre
   E deviation of the eyes to the side of the auditory meatus irrigated with ice cold water

12.13 Which of the following may be mistaken for childhood or infantile seizures:
   A reflex anoxic episodes
   B Romano-Ward syndrome
   C night terrors
   D masturbation
   E breath holding episodes

12.14 Which of the following visual field defects are correctly paired with the neuroanatomical lesion:
   A homonymous hemianopia: craniopharyngioma at the optic chiasma
   B absent pupillary response in one eye: lesion of lateral geniculate body
   C bitemporal hemianopia: unilateral optic radiation lesion
   D quadrantic homonymous field defect: parietal lobe lesion
   E 'tunnel' vision: optic nerve lesion

12.10	A	False	Such seizures present before puberty and require a
	B	False	pathognomonic supportive EEG. Rarely they may
	C	True	develop into generalized seizures. Most absences
	D	False	respond to valproate or ethosuximide. There is
	E	False	rarely any obvious underlying cortical focal abnormality.

12.11	A	True	Infantile spasms usually indicate a severe underlying
	B	True	intracranial abnormality. Most children manifest
	C	False	psychomotor retardation. Treatment has depended
	D	False	upon steroids or ACTH. The EEG usually shows
	E	True	hypsarrhythmia.

12.12	A	False	Brainstem death criteria do not apply to the preterm
	B	False	infant. Fixed dilated pupils, in the presence of
	C	False	hypothermia, do not indicate brain death.
	D	True	Phenobarbitone and other sedatives must not have
	E	False	been recently given prior to testing for brainstem death. Deviation of the eyes towards the side irrigated with ice cold water indicates an intact brainstem.

12.13	A	True	All the above may initially be mistaken for seizures.
	B	True	Romano Ward syndrome is an arrhythmia
	C	True	associated with a prolonged QT pattern on the ECG.
	D	True	
	E	True	

12.14	A	False	Unilateral blindness usually represents optic nerve
	B	False	dysfunction whilst tunnel vision is more commonly
	C	False	associated with hysterical phenomena. Chiasmal
	D	True	lesions result in bitemporal hemianopias. A
	E	False	homonymous hemianopia implies a lesion posterior to the chiasma in the optic tract or the optic radiation. Lesions in the latter may be a quadrantic field defect. The lateral geniculate body is the site of the convergence of the optic tracts and the dispersion of the optic radiations. Pupillary responses are only affected when fibres proximal to the lateral geniculate body in the midbrain or 3rd nerve are damaged.

12.15 Results of cord hemisection include:
- A contralateral paralysis
- B contralateral loss of sensation
- C loss of ipsilateral position sense
- D diplegia
- E hypoglossal paralysis

12.16 Features of the anterior spinal artery syndrome include:
- A preservation of muscle activity
- B loss of vibratory sense
- C preservation of position sense
- D loss of pain sensation
- E loss of temperature sensation

12.17 Third cranial nerve palsy includes:
- A partial ptosis
- B pupillary dilatation
- C microphthalmos
- D superior rotation of the eye
- E adducted eye position

12.18 The following are correct statements regarding the innervation of the upper limb:
- A median nerve innervates thumb flexion
- B radial nerve innervates the interosseous nerves
- C ulnar nerve supinates the forearm
- D ulnar sensory loss includes the 4th and 5th fingers
- E radial neuropathy results in wrist drop

12.19 Which of the following cerebrospinal fluid laboratory results are correctly paired with their clinical entities:
- A neutrophil count 20 000/mm^3: tuberculous meningitis
- B protein 4 g/l: viral encephalitis
- C CSF glucose 0.9 mmol/l: mumps, meningoencephalitis
- D low CSF chloride: tuberculous meningitis
- E CSF glucose/blood glucose ratio of 0.40: bacterial meningitis

12.15 A **False**   Cord hemisection (Brown-Séquard syndrome)
       B **True**   results in ipsilateral paralysis and contralateral loss
       C **False**   of sensory signs.
       D **False**
       E **False**

12.16 A **False**   The anterior spinal artery supplies the entire cord
       B **False**   except for the dorsal columns. Thus position and
       C **True**   vibratory sense is preserved but paralysis is present,
       D **True**   and pain and temperature senses are lost.
       E **True**

12.17 A **False**   Third nerve palsies manifest as complete ptosis,
       B **True**   pupil dilatation with a divergent strabismus (eye is
       C **False**   'down and out').
       D **False**
       E **False**

12.18 A **True**   The **median nerve** supplies: **forearm** (pronator,
       B **False**   wrist abduction and radial flexion); **hand** (thumb
       C **False**   movements, index and middle finger flexion and first
       D **True**   two lumbricals). **Sensory** loss involves the thumb
       E **True**   and first two fingers.
                      The **ulnar nerve** supplies: **forearm** (ulnar wrist
                      flexion); **hand** (4th/5th flexion, 5th abduction and
                      opposition, interosseous muscles, 3rd/4th
                      lumbricales and thumb adduction). **Sensory** loss
                      over the 4th and 5th fingers.
                      The **radial nerve** supplies: **forearm** (supinator,
                      extensors). **Sensory** loss is over the back of the
                      hand.

12.19 A **False**   The CSF picture of a bacterial meningitis is of a high
       B **False**   neutrophil count associated with an elevated protein
       C **True**   level and low glucose concentration with a CSF/
       D **True**   blood glucose ratio of not less than 0.6. TB
       E **True**   meningitis is associated with an elevated
                      lymphocyte count. Massive CSF protein
                      concentrations are not usually elevated in viral
                      encephalitis. Low CSF glucose levels are unusual in
                      viral meningitis except mumps.

12.20 Features of Friedreich's ataxia include:
- A prominent deep reflexes
- B pes cavus
- C extensor plantar response
- D steatorrhoea
- E dysarthria

12.21 The following are true of the Guillain-Barré syndrome:
- A it is associated with a symmetrical flaccid paralysis
- B progression of the disease for several weeks is common
- C sensory symptoms are absent
- D muscle tenderness excludes the diagnosis
- E CSF analysis reveals a high cell count but normal CSF biochemistry

12.22 Duchenne muscular dystrophy:
- A is autosomal dominant
- B is due to excess cellular dystrophin
- C results from a single point mutation in the gene intron
- D presents after the age of 8 years
- E is confirmed by the pathognomonic Gower sign

12.23 Prion diseases:
- A are caused by viruses
- B are transmissible proteins
- C include Creutzfeldt-Jakob disease
- D result from neuronal accumulation of prion protein
- E include subacute sclerosing panencephalitis

12.24 Features of cerebral palsy diplegia include:
- A toe walking
- B scissoring
- C hip flexion
- D external rotation of legs
- E poor balance

12.20   A False   Friedreich's ataxia is a cause of progressive ataxia
        B True   with the following features: ataxia; loss of vibration/
        C True   position sense; absent deep tendon reflexes;
        D False   extensor plantars; nystagmus; dysarthria; pes cavus;
        E True   kyphoscoliosis; cardiac conduction defects; and
                     increased incidence of diabetes mellitus.
                     Steatorrhoea is a feature of abetalipoproteinaemia,
                     another cause of chronic ataxia.

12.21   A True   The Guillain-Barré syndrome manifests as an
        B False   ascending areflexic flaccid paralysis with minimal
        C False   sensory involvement. The disease is usually acute
        D False   with progression over the first few days. Respiratory
        E False   involvement may occur. CSF analysis reveals
                     increased CSF protein levels without associated cell
                     count.

12.22   A False   Duchenne muscular dystrophy is an X-linked
        B False   disorder occurring in 1:4000 live male births.
        C False   Presentation is usually in infancy. The Gower sign
        D False   of rising by 'walking up the legs' occurs but is not
        E False   pathognomonic. The basic pathology is an absence
                     of the cell membrane protein, dystrophin. The
                     genetic defect is one of several point mutations,
                     deletions or duplications in the exons of this very
                     large gene.

12.23   A False   Prion diseases are believed to result from the
        B True   intraneuronal accumulation of abnormal
        C True   transmissible proteins. They are not viral. Subacute
        D True   sclerosing panencephalitis is a result of previous
        E False   and possibly chronic CNS measles infection.

12.24   A True   Pre- or perinatal causes often account for a spastic
        B True   diplegia. The characteristic features include
        C True   increased adduction and flexion at the hip giving rise
        D False   to scissoring. Shortening of the Achilles tendon
        E True   results in tip-toe walking. Internal rotation of the legs
                     is common. Balance is often precarious.

12.25 Rett syndrome:
  A predominantly affects boys
  B manifests in the neonatal period
  C is suggested by autistic mannerisms
  D has a pathognomonic EEG abnormality
  E has X-linked inheritance

12.25 A **False**   Rett syndrome predominates in girls (1:15 000).
       B **False**   Early development is normal but problems manifest
       C **True**   about 18 months to 2 years. Autistic features often
       D **False**   predominate. It is a progressive problem. EEG
       E **False**   abnormalities occur but are not diagnostic. Cortical
                      atrophy does occur but the aetiology remains
                      unclear.

13. Psychosocial paediatrics

13.1 Which of the following statements concerning chronic fatigue syndrome are correct:
- A clinical depression is a universal feature on psychological testing
- B features may be precipitated by infectious mononucleosis
- C outcome is related to acceptance of psychosomatic disturbance
- D easy fatiguability is very common
- E myalgia excludes the diagnosis

13.2 Anorexia nervosa:
- A has an improved outcome in affected boys
- B may be associated with metabolic disturbance
- C is associated with precocious puberty
- D is often associated with disturbed family dynamics
- E is treated with appetite stimulants

13.3 Depression in children:
- A has a female preponderance
- B is rarely accompanied by a family history of depression
- C is not associated with an increased risk of suicide
- D usually responds to cognitive-behaviour therapy
- E predominates in the prepubertal child

13.4 'Munchausen by proxy' syndrome:
- A is more common in medical or paramedical professionals
- B may simulate apnoea
- C is usually committed by the mother
- D is more common in depressed parents
- E is more common in parents who are prohibited-drug misusers

13.5 Adolescent drug abuse:
- A is more common in girls
- B is rarely associated with eating disorders in affected girls
- C is associated with teenage pregnancy
- D may be a feature of family dysfunction
- E is associated with parasuicide

13.1 A **False**   Chronic fatigue syndrome remains controversial
      B **True**   both in diagnosis, pathophysiology and treatment.
      C **True**   Easy fatiguability is common. Somatic features may
      D **True**   be common, e.g. recurrent fevers, but are generally
      E **False**   mild. Fever does not exceed 38.5°C. Myalgia is
                       common. Many cases seem to be precipitated by
                       infections including EBV. Sufferers who concentrate
                       purely on the physical aspects of CFS seem to fare
                       worse than those who accept the psychological
                       facets of the illness.

13.2 A **False**   Anorexia and other eating disorders are often
      B **True**   features of disturbed family life. Some may be
      C **False**   bulimic with vomiting sufficient to cause electrolyte
      D **True**   abnormalities. Many girls suffer pubertal delay. Boys
      E **False**   are usually more affected than girls and thus have a
                       poorer prognosis. Appetite stimulants are rarely
                       used.

13.3 A **True**   Depressive illness has an equal sex ratio in those
      B **False**   below 10 years of age but a female predominance
      C **False**   after that. One-third have an affected parent and
      D **True**   suicide is a definite risk problem. The teenage years
      E **False**   are the most likely to be affected. Cognitive-
                       behaviour therapy concentrates on identifying,
                       changing and monitoring learnt, negative thoughts,
                       e.g. of low self-esteem.

13.4 A **True**   Most of such acts are committed by the chief carer
      B **True**   and often the mother. There is an increased risk if
      C **True**   the carer was in a medical career or one allied to the
      D **True**   caring professions. Suffocation may simulate
      E **False**   apnoea and only become recognized during covert
                       surveillance. Parental depression is common
                       although parental drug-misuse does not seem to be
                       of such relevance in the majority of cases.

13.5 A **False**   Adolescent drug abuse is more common in males. It
      B **False**   is associated with suicide, deliberate self-harm,
      C **True**   unwanted pregnancy and sexually transmitted
      D **True**   infections.
      E **True**

14. Children's Act

14.1 Duties invoked by the 1989 Act include:
- A to provide preschool education for those under 5
- B to keep a register of disabled children
- C to provide family centres
- D to provide day care facilities for the under 5s
- E to promote contact between children and their families

14.2 Which of the following are correct statements regarding child protection issues:
- A a child assessment order is indicated if the child has suffered recent injury
- B a child assessment order lasts for 7 days
- C an emergency protection order lasts for 7 days
- D an emergency protection order can only be ordered by the courts
- E a recovery order is issued if a child is deemed to be in danger

14.1 A False   The main issues of the Children's Act 1989 include
      B True   the paramountcy of the child whose welfare must be
      C True   considered in all cases. Children should be safe and
      D True   delay minimized in dealing with problems. Children
      E True   must be given information and the right to help in
                determining their future. Parents should be helped to
                look after their children. Preschool education for
                children not in need is not a feature.

14.2 A False   A child assessment order is used if a child is at risk
      B True   of significant harm but not at immediate risk. It lasts
      C False   for a maximum of 7 days. An emergency protection
      D True   order lasts for 8 days and may be renewed for a
      E False   further 7 days. It enables a child to be made safe
                when at risk of immediate harm. It is made by the
                courts. A recovery order, made by the court, is when
                a child in care has been deemed unlawfully kept
                away from the responsible carer.

15. Rheumatology and orthopaedics

15.1 **Pauciarticular juvenile chronic arthritis:**
  A is usually rheumatoid factor seropositive
  B is classically HLA B27 related
  C is an erosive large joint disease
  D may be complicated by iritis if antinuclear factor seronegative
  E usually requires immunosuppressive therapy

15.2 **Which of the following are recognized complications of Henoch-Schönlein purpura:**
  A splenic sequestration
  B acute intussusception
  C proteinuria
  D coronary arteritis
  E scrotal pain

15.3 **Perthes disease:**
  A is most common in the peripubertal boy
  B results from avascular necrosis
  C is most frequently unilateral in distribution
  D results from an undertreated osteomyelitis
  E presents as an acutely painful limp

15.4 **Which of the following are causes of a painful limp:**
  A slipped femoral epiphyses
  B Duchenne muscular dystrophy
  C Gaucher's disease
  D irritable hip
  E Osgood-Schlatter disease

15.1 A **False**   Pauciarticular juvenile chronic arthritis is a large joint
      B **False**   disorder affecting four or less joints. It is rheumatoid
      C **False**   seronegative but often antinuclear (ANA)
      D **False**   seropositive. If ANA positive, slit light examination is
      E **False**   mandatory as iritis commonly complicates this
                    clinical picture. The disease is rarely erosive and
                    does not require immunosuppressive therapy.
                    Symptomatic treatment with non-steroidal anti-
                    inflammatory medication is usually sufficient.

15.2 A **False**   Henoch-Schönlein purpura is the most common
      B **True**   cause of non-thrombocytopenic purpura. It is a
      C **True**   vasculitis associated with circulating immune
      D **False**   complexes, often of IgA type. Intussusception,
      E **True**   abdominal pain and gastrointestinal haemorrhage
                    are common gut complications. Haematuria and
                    proteinuria occur in 60% but gross proteinuria is rare
                    and renal manifestations may persist for a
                    considerable time. Scrotal pain may be due to
                    vasculitis progressing to torsion. Coronary arteritis is
                    a feature of Kawasaki's disease. Splenic
                    sequestration occurs in sickle cell disease.

15.3 A **False**   Perthes disease occurs in the age range of 4–8
      B **True**   years. 10% of cases are bilateral. The underlying
      C **True**   pathology is avascular necrosis of the femoral head
      D **False**   and not osteomyelitis. Presentation is usually
      E **False**   insidious with a relatively painless limp. The pain
                    may be referred to the knee. Radiological evidence
                    of femoral head flattening may indicate the need for
                    surgical osteotomy.

15.4 A **True**   Irritable hip is a common cause for a painful limp. It
      B **False**   is probably postviral in nature. These symptoms
      C **True**   may be mimicked by the nonspecific coxalgia
      D **True**   associated with Gaucher's disease. Osgood-
      E **True**   Schlatter disease is due to inflammation or avulsion
                    of the tibial tuberosity.

15.5 **Which of the following statements regarding bacterial osteomyelitis are correct:**
A the erythrocyte sedimentation rate (ESR) is the most rapid acute phase reactant to resolve with successful treatment
B Haemophilus species are the most common infecting organism in those with haemoglobinopathies
C group B haemolytic streptococci remain important causes of neonatal osteomyelitis
D surgical intervention is always necessary in neonatal osteomyelitis
E bone scans are never positive in the absence of radiological abnormalities

15.6 **Sarcoidosis:**
A most commonly presents with ophthalmic involvement
B is associated with elevated angiotensin converting enzyme level
C is best diagnosed using the Kveim test
D is associated with hypogammaglobulinaemia
E rarely causes chest X-ray changes in affected children

15.7 **Features of neonatal lupus include:**
A thrombocytopenia
B congenital heart block
C anti-Ro autoantibodies present in mother
D positive anti-ds DNA antibodies in the infant
E hepatosplenomegaly

15.8 **Dermatomyositis:**
A has a prevalence of 1:1000 children
B is commonly associated with malignancy in adults and children
C causes early muscle calcinosis
D results in positive antinuclear antibodies
E is associated with an abnormal electromyogram

15.5	A	**False**	Staphylococci remain the most common causative organisms except during the neonatal period when group B streptococci, enterococci and coliforms are important aetiologies. Salmonellae have a predilection for those with sickle cell haemoglobinopathy. Whilst the ESR is an important acute phase marker, the C-reactive protein estimation remains the more sensitive reactant showing earlier response to infection and treatment than the ESR. Many neonatal osteomyelitis infections do not require surgery. Bone scans may identify infection before standard X-rays.
	B	**False**	
	C	**True**	
	D	**False**	
	E	**False**	
15.6	A	**True**	Sarcoidosis is rare in children. The most common presentations are either eye signs or non-tender lymphadenopathy. The chest X-ray is usually abnormal. CD4 lymphopenia is common. Hypergammaglobulinaemia is the usual pattern in over 50% of patients. Angiotensin converting enzyme levels are elevated in pulmonary sarcoid but this may occur in other diseases. The intradermal Kveim test, using an extract of sarcoid tissue, is largely unhelpful requiring a biopsy 6 weeks later. False positives occur and a negative test is unhelpful.
	B	**True**	
	C	**False**	
	D	**False**	
	E	**False**	
15.7	A	**True**	Classic features include: macular-papular rash; heart block; hepatosplenomegaly; thrombocytopenia; and autoimmune haemolytic anaemia. Maternal anti-Ro antibody is associated with congenital heart block. Neither rheumatoid factor nor anti-ds DNA are usually detected in the infant.
	B	**True**	
	C	**True**	
	D	**False**	
	E	**True**	
15.8	A	**False**	Prevalence is approximately 2 per million. Associated malignancy occurs in 20% of adults but is extremely rarely in children. Calcinosis is a late finding. Other features include: oedema; Gottron's papules; vasculitic ulcers; and abnormal muscle biochemistry and electrophysiological function. ANA is usually negative. Presenting features are often proximal muscle weakness and the purple skin heliotrope facial rash.
	B	**False**	
	C	**False**	
	D	**False**	
	E	**True**	

Rheumatology and orthopaedics

15.9 The following microbiological agents are known to cause arthralgia:
A rubella
B mycoplasma
C yersinia
D parvovirus
E chlamydia

15.10 The following are recognized features of psoriatic arthritis in childhood:
A peak age of 4 years
B nail pitting precedes arthritis
C male predominance
D erosive joint disease affecting large joints
E seronegativity

15.11 Which of the following statements concerning osteogenesis imperfecta is correct:
A all affected children have blue-coloured sclerae
B some affected fetuses are stillborn
C aortic root connective tissue disease may complicate certain types
D the basic defect is probably aberrant collagen hydroxylation
E inheritance is usually autosomal dominant

15.12 Arthrogryphosis multiplex congenita:
A is a defect in distal bone mineralization
B causes limb reduction defects
C is usually lethal
D is characteristically associated with mental retardation
E may have a myopathic aetiology

15.9 A True   A wide range of organisms may cause both
      B True   arthralgia and arthritis. This may be due to direct
      C True   infection or by a post-infection immune response
      D True   often termed a 'reactive arthritis'.
      E True

15.10 A False   Psoriatic arthropathy is a seronegative arthritis
      B False   which is usually non-erosive. The peak age affected
      C False   is 10 years. There is a female preponderance and
      D False   often a family history of psoriasis. Whilst large joints
      E True   may be affected, small joints, particularly the
                 interphalangeal joints, are commonly involved. Other
                 features of psoriasis may develop after the arthritis
                 in some cases.

15.11 A False   Osteogenesis imperfecta is a heterogenous group of
      B True   disorders of collagen synthesis. The underlying
      C True   defect seems to be overhydroxylation of α (1) chain
      D True   collagen. Incidence may be either autosomal
      E False   dominant or recessive and prevalence is 1:10 000–
                 50 000. 80% of cases are type I. Type II is often
                 lethal in the perinatal period. Blue sclerae may be
                 absent in types III and IV. Dentinogenesis imperfecta
                 may coexist.

15.12 A False   Arthrogryphosis multiplex congenita is a complex of
      B False   signs rather than a diagnostic entity. Clinically the
      C False   infant may have multiple limb contractures with
      D False   normal underlying skeletal pattern. The contractures
      E True   may, however, cause joint dislocations and fixed
                 deformities, e.g. talipes equinovarus. Neuropathic
                 and myopathic causes may be apparent but usually
                 there is no obvious cause. Treatment is orthopaedic
                 with physiotherapy. Mental retardation is not a
                 common association. Occasionally it may be
                 associated with a neural tube defect, trisomy or
                 maternal muscular disease.

15.13 **Achondroplasia:**
- A is a cause of proportionate short stature
- B has an autosomal dominant inheritance
- C causes relative macrocephaly
- D is associated with deformities of the hand
- E is associated with increased frequency of long-bone fractures

15.14 **Osteosarcoma:**
- A has a peak incidence in the prepubertal child
- B exhibits the 'sunray spicule' radiological feature
- C is more commonly found in the ends of long bones
- D usually presents as a pathological fracture
- E metastasizes early in the disease

15.15 **Which of the following autoantibodies are correctly paired with the corresponding disease:**
- A double-stranded DNA: systemic lupus erythematosus
- B anti-smooth muscle: chronic active hepatitis
- C anti-centromere: dermatomyositis
- D anti-neutrophil cytoplasmic antibody (ANCA): Behçet's disease
- E antiribonucleic protein: mixed connective tissue disease

15.13 A **False**   Achondroplasia causes disproportionate short
       B **True**   stature. Endochondral bone formation is defective
       C **True**   whereas membranous bone formation is normal.
       D **True**   Therefore the vault of the skull (membranous
       E **False**   ossification) occurs at a normal rate compared to the
                       base of the skull giving rise to the relative
                       macrocephaly. Whilst inheritance is autosomal
                       dominant, most are new mutations. There is often a
                       marked lumbar lordosis together with a thoracic
                       kyphosis. The hands are short with the fingers
                       similar in length. their lack of full adduction gives rise
                       to the 'trident' hand deformity.

15.14 A **False**   This malignancy has a male sex preponderance
       B **True**   affecting post or late pubertal ages. Typical
       C **True**   presentation is a painful swelling at the ends of a
       D **False**   long bone. It is a fast growing tumour which
       E **True**   metastasizes early to the lungs and other bony sites.
                       It may be seen as a second tumour in those with
                       familial retinoblastoma. X-ray appearances include
                       spicules of new bone, periosteal formation and
                       osteolytic lesions. 80% of relapses are pulmonary.

15.15 A **True**   Anti-centromere antibodies occur in 70–90% of
       B **True**   cases of CREST syndrome. ANCA occur in more
       C **False**   than 90% of cases of Wegener's granulomatosis.
       D **False**
       E **True**

16. Statistics

16.1 **Which of the following statements regarding measures of central value is correct:**
    A median is the measurement that occurs most frequently
    B mode is the measurement that occurs most frequently
    C mean is the measurement that occurs most frequently
    D variance is the measurement that occurs most frequently
    E range is the average series of measurements encountered

16.2 **The following are measures of dispersion:**
    A standard deviation
    B coefficient of variation
    C variance
    D standard error of the means
    E range

16.3 **Which of the following are tests of probability:**
    A Student's T test
    B Chi-Square test
    C Mann-Whitney U test
    D Wilcoxon's signed rank test
    E coefficient of correlation

16.4 **Features of a normal (Gaussian) distribution include:**
    A more observations at the extremes of measurement
    B symmetrical bell shape
    C one standard deviation either side of the mean includes 68% of the population
    D mean and mode but not median are the same value
    E mean, mode and median are the same value

16.5 **The following statistical statements are correct:**
    A standard error is calculated by dividing the standard deviation of the sample by the square root of the number of observations in the sample
    B an inevitable event is given the probability denoted p=0.5
    C a p value of 0.01 is insignificant
    D complete correlation has a coefficient of 1
    E non-parametric tests of probability are used for data which is not normally distributed

16.1	A	**False**	Mode is the value most frequently encountered.
	B	**True**	Median is the central value when the series of
	C	**False**	values are arranged in order. The mean is the
	D	**False**	mathematical average.
	E	**False**	

16.2	A	**True**	Range is the difference between the highest and
	B	**True**	lowest values observed. Variance is the sum of the
	C	**True**	squares of the deviations from the mean divided by
	D	**True**	the number of observations. Its coefficient is the
	E	**True**	standard deviation expressed as a percentage of the mean. Standard deviation is the square root of the variance. Standard error of the means is the standard deviation of means around the population mean.

16.3	A	**True**	Student's T test and Chi-Square are parametric
	B	**True**	tests. The others are non-parametric tests.
	C	**True**	
	D	**True**	
	E	**False**	

16.4	A	**False**	Gaussian distribution includes more measurements
	B	**True**	around the mean. Mean, mode and median are all
	C	**True**	the same value.
	D	**False**	
	E	**True**	

16.5	A	**True**	P=1 when an event is inevitable. P values less than
	B	**False**	0.05 are significant.
	C	**False**	
	D	**True**	
	E	**True**	

17. Pharmacology

17.1 Lamotrigine:
- A is the treatment of choice for status epilepticus
- B is contraindicated in generalized seizures
- C is a GABA transaminase inhibitor
- D reduces glutamate release
- E is excreted by the gut

17.2 The macrolide antibiotics:
- A include azithromycin
- B are only bacteriostatic
- C inhibit microsomal protein synthesis
- D penetrate tissues poorly
- E result in a toxic interaction with terfenadine

17.3 Which of the following are anticonvulsants:
- A vigabatrin
- B paraldehyde
- C clonazepam
- D temazepam
- E gabapentin

17.4 Cisapride:
- A is a prokinetic agent
- B is an anti-*Helicobacter pylori* treatment
- C increases the resting tone of the gastro-oesophageal sphincter
- D reduces gastric acid secretion
- E may cause constipation

17.5 Proposed mechanisms of action of exogenous surfactants include:
- A reduction in intrapulmonary water
- B reduction in pulmonary vascular pressure
- C inotropic effect on myocardial function
- D direct anti-cytokine role in the alveoli
- E increased surfactant precursor pool

17.1 A **False**   Lamotrigine, a new anticonvulsant, acts at the
      B **False**   sodium channel and reduces glutamate release. It is
      C **False**   of benefit as add-on therapy in partial seizures and
      D **True**   secondary generalized seizures. It is predominantly
      E **False**   renally excreted.

17.2 A **True**   The macrolides include erythromycin, clarithromycin
      B **False**   and azithromycin. They penetrate tissues well and
      C **True**   are both bacteriostatic and bacteriocidal depending
      D **False**   on the organism. Erythromycin and clarithromycin
      E **True**   may cause arrhythmias if given with terfenadine.

17.3 A **True**
      B **True**
      C **True**
      D **False**
      E **True**

17.4 A **True**   Cisapride increases gut emptying thus resulting in
      B **False**   diarrhoea. It alters sphincter tone but has no effect
      C **True**   on gastric acid secretion.
      D **False**
      E **False**

17.5 A **False**   Surfactants seem to have several beneficial
      B **True**   properties. Immediate benefits seen may be due to
      C **False**   an effect on pulmonary vascular pressure rather
      D **False**   than surface tension lowering properties.
      E **True**

Pharmacology

17.6 Which of the following drugs are correctly paired with the sign of overdose toxicity:
- A amytriptyline: heart block
- B aspirin: dilated pupils
- C desferrioxamine: hypotension
- D sumatriptan: chest pain
- E paracetamol: tachypnoea

17.7 Pizotifen:
- A is an anti-arrhythmic agent
- B is a membrane stabilizing agent
- C is used in the treatment of abdominal migraine
- D causes sedation
- E may cause weight gain

17.8 Which of the following statements regarding pharmacokinetics are true:
- A pharmacokinetics explains the effects of drugs on the metabolism
- B clearance values represent the theoretical volume of fluid from which the drug is completely removed in a given time
- C volume of distribution equals the circulating volume
- D bioavailability describes the proportion of the drug appearing in the circulation protein bound
- E non-linear kinetics accounts for large changes in concentration following small increases in dose

17.9 Correct statements regarding diuretics include:
- A thiazides are loop diuretics
- B thiazides are potassium sparing diuretics
- C thiazides rely on excretion into the renal tubules
- D thiazides may cause hypercalcaemia
- E frusemide has smooth muscle relaxing properties

17.10 Which of the following antibiotics are correctly paired with their usual spectrum of activity or sensitive organism:
- A erythromycin: mycoplasma species
- B ceftibuten: Gram-negative pathogens
- C ciprofloxacin: pseudomonas
- D clarithromycin: atypical mycobacteria
- E ciprofloxacin: campylobacter

17.11 Drugs contraindicated during pregnancy include:
- A cotrimoxazole
- B carbimazole
- C enalapril
- D paracetamol
- E etretinate

17.6 A **True**   Aspirin poisoning causes tachypnoea due to
      B **False**   alkalosis before subsequent metabolic acidosis.
      C **True**   Tricyclic antidepressants may cause either
      D **True**   tachyarrhythmias or heart block. Sumatriptan,
      E **False**   an antimigraine, may cause chest pain and angina
                      as it causes vasospasm.

17.7 A **False**   Pizotifen is an anti-migraine medication also of
      B **False**   benefit in abdominal migraine. It is a serotonin
      C **True**   antagonist.
      D **True**
      E **True**

17.8 A **False**   Pharmacokinetics describes what the body does to a
      B **True**   drug. Volume of distribution is the volume that would
      C **False**   accommodate all the drug if its concentration was
      D **False**   the same as in plasma. Bioavailability includes only
      E **True**   free drug.

17.9 A **False**   Thiazides are weak diuretics. They may cause
      B **False**   increased calcium reabsorption.
      C **True**
      D **True**
      E **True**

17.10 A **True**
      B **True**
      C **True**
      D **True**
      E **True**

17.11 A **False**   Although cotrimoxazole has a potential teratogenic
      B **True**   effect as trimethoprim is a folate antagonist, it is not
      C **True**   absolutely contraindicated. Carbimazole may cause
      D **False**   hypothyroidism and neonatal goitre. Enalapril and
      E **True**   other ACE inhibitors may affect fetal renal function
                      and cause oligohydramnios. Etretinate is
                      teratogenic.

17.12 Pharmacological treatments of persistent pulmonary hypertension of the neonate include:
A magnesium sulphate infusion
B tolazoline infusion
C frusemide
D prostacyclin infusion
E indomethacin

17.13 Which of the following asthma devices is appropriate for the corresponding age group:
A metered dose inhaler: 4–7 year olds
B metered dose inhaler with large volume spacer: less than 2 year olds
C diskhaler: 2–4 year olds
D turbohaler: 7–10 year olds
E spinhalers: less than 2 years

17.14 Features of drug administration in the neonate include:
A higher volume of distribution
B increased membrane permeability
C increased protein binding
D decreased glucuronidation
E decreased glomerular filtration of drugs

17.15 Pharmacological effects of glucocorticoids include:
A reduction in gluconeogenesis
B suppression of arachidonic acid metabolism
C enhanced distal tubule reabsorption of sodium
D decreased gastric acid secretion
E increased renal calcium loss

17.16 Potential uses for inhaled steroid therapy include:
A chronic asthma
B acute laryngotracheobronchitis
C chronic lung disease of the newborn
D post-bronchiolitis inflammation
E bronchial hyperresponsiveness

17.17 Adenosine:
A is of benefit in ventricular tachyarrhythmias
B is the drug of choice for supraventricular tachycardia
C is given as a slow infusion
D has a half life of 30 minutes
E may cause prolonged hypotension

17.12	A	**True**	Neonatal pulmonary hypertension may be relieved by vasodilators such as tolazoline or prostacyclin. Hypotension is a major complication. Magnesium is a smooth muscle relaxant.
	B	**True**	
	C	**False**	
	D	**True**	
	E	**False**	

17.13	A	**False**	Generally inhaled therapy must be via a spacer until at least 4 years of age. Dry powder inhalers may be of benefit after this age depending on the child's ability and that of the parent. Metered dose inhalers alone should not be prescribed to those below 12 years.
	B	**True**	
	C	**False**	
	D	**True**	
	E	**False**	

17.14	A	**False**	Volume of distribution is a feature of the drug. Increased lipid permeability is noted. Glucuronidation in the liver is reduced.
	B	**True**	
	C	**False**	
	D	**True**	
	E	**True**	

17.15	A	**False**
	B	**True**
	C	**True**
	D	**False**
	E	**True**

17.16	A	**True**	All of the above are potential uses of inhaled steroids although many are not licensed indications at present.
	B	**True**	
	C	**True**	
	D	**True**	
	E	**True**	

17.17	A	**False**	Adenosine is used as a treatment for supraventricular tachycardia. It is given into a large vein, preferably draining into the superior vena cava, as a fast bolus. The half life is only a few seconds. Hypotension is a side-effect of verapamil therapy.
	B	**True**	
	C	**False**	
	D	**False**	
	E	**False**	

17.18 DNase therapy in cystic fibrosis:
- A utilizes animal derived enzyme
- B is associated with a high incidence of anaphylaxis
- C is given intravenously
- D reduces sputum viscoelasticity
- E replaces the need for physiotherapy

17.19 Which of the following are antiviral medications:
- A ribavirin
- B ganciclovir
- C famciclovir
- D inosine pranobex
- E foscarnet

17.20 Which of the following should be avoided in renal impairment:
- A gentamicin
- B nitrofurantoin
- C acyclovir
- D ranitidine
- E erythromycin

17.18 A **False**   DNase is a nebulized recombinant enzyme which
       B **False**   reduces the thickness of sputum in those with cystic
       C **False**   fibrosis. The optimal indications for use are still
       D **True**   uncertain.
       E **False**

17.19 A **True**   All are antiviral agents. Ribavirin has a role in both
       B **True**   bronchiolitis and some viral haemorrhagic fevers.
       C **True**   Ganciclovir and foscarnet are anti-CMV drugs with
       D **True**   foscarnet of value in CMV retinitis. Famciclovir is
       E **True**   similar to acyclovir. Inosine has been used in the
                       treatment of herpes simplex.

17.20 A **True**
       B **True**
       C **True**
       D **True**
       E **True**

18. Respirology

18.1 **The following statements apply in bronchiolitis:**
    A most cases are seen in the autumn and winter months
    B Chlamydia is a recognized causative organism in children under 12 weeks of age
    C preterm infants with chronic lung disease are not at high risk
    D hypoxia is not a feature in the acute phase
    E treatment with corticosteroids often shortens the course of the disease

18.2 **The following statements regarding the lungs in acquired immunodeficiency syndrome (AIDS) are correct:**
    A most patients develop *Pneumocystis carinii* pneumonia
    B bronchial lavage fluid contains large amounts of neutrophils
    C inhaled pentamidine is used in the treatment of *Pneumocystis pneumonia*
    D lymphocytic interstitial pneumonitis is a recognized feature
    E pleural effusions commonly occur in affected children

18.3 **The following are true of pulmonary complications of inhalation:**
    A the child presents with signs and symptoms of lower respiratory tract infection
    B milk inhalation is a common problem in infancy
    C children with neuromuscular problems are more at risk
    D bronchospasm is rarely a problem
    E tracheal aspirate shows fat laden macrophages

18.1 A **True**   Bronchiolitis commonly affects infants where there
      B **True**   are features suggestive of a viral illness, e.g. coryza,
      C **False** cough, fever. The infants are often dyspnoeic and
      D **False** tachypnoeic. The work of breathing rapidly increases
      E **False** with the progress of the disease. Chest retraction
                   with wheezing are common findings on clinical
                   examination. Feeding difficulties occur. The infants
                   become lethargic and dehydrated due to vomiting.
                   There are non-specific changes seen on the chest
                   X-ray. Good nursing care and observation are
                   essential in the management of these patients.
                   Ribavirin has been used when RSV has been
                   isolated in the high-risk patients, e.g. infants with
                   chronic lung disease or congenital heart disease,
                   preterm infants with chronic lung disease.

18.2 A **True**   Lung involvement in AIDS is a recognized
      B **False** complication. The respiratory symptoms are often
      C **True**   insidious. Other opportunistic organisms such as
      D **True**   *CMV, Mycobacterium avium* and *Mycobacterium*
      E **False** *tuberculosis* cause troublesome problems.
                   Corticosteroids have been used to relieve hypoxia.
                   Co-trimoxazole in high doses has been used in the
                   treatment of pneumonia.

18.3 A **True**   This clinical problem is often underdiagnosed.
      B **True**   Inhalation of food occurs as a result of disorders of
      C **True**   sucking and swallowing, oesophageal
      D **False** malfunctioning resulting in the food getting back into
      E **True**   the pharynx, or abnormal communications between
                   the airways and the oesophagus. These children
                   have respiratory symptoms and often vomit during or
                   soon after feeds. Radiological changes seen depend
                   on the age of the child and presence or absence of
                   secondary infection. Antibiotics are indicated if there
                   is secondary infection.

18.4 **The following statements about apparent life-threatening events (ALTE) are correct:**
  A they are seen in both preterm infants and term infants
  B gastro-oesophageal reflux may be causative
  C a change in the pattern of bowel movements may herald an attack
  D preterm infants are at greater risk of a second event
  E pertussis is a recognized cause

18.5 **The following mechanisms have been identified in asthma:**
  A histamine is released by the inflammatory cells acting on the smooth muscles
  B structural changes are seen in chronic asthmatic patients
  C mast cells and neutrophils have no biological role in the pathogenesis of asthma
  D plasma leak and oedema do not occur in the bronchial muscle wall
  E viral infections are recognized precipitating factors in the inflammatory process

18.6 **The following are correct statements regarding acute bronchiolitis:**
  A in 75% of cases respiratory syncytial virus (RSV) is responsible
  B hyponatraemia is a complication in the acute phase of the illness
  C bronchodilator therapy significantly improves the symptoms
  D bronchial hyperresponsiveness is common after the illness
  E the spread is mainly by droplets from infants and adults

18.4 A **True**   An apparent life-threatening event is also known as
      B **True**   near miss sudden infant death syndrome. These
      C **False**   infants present for medical care shortly after the
      D **True**   event where a combination of pallor, cyanosis,
      E **True**   apnoea, bradycardia, hypertonia or hypotonia have
                      been observed. In a large proportion of cases the
                      cause is not known. Infections such as RSV and
                      pertussis, cardiac arrhythmias, and central nervous
                      system disorders have been diagnosed in some of
                      the infants after the event. Detailed enquiry into the
                      event is essential. A brief period of admission and
                      investigations are appropriate. Some of the infants
                      may be left with neurodevelopment delay.
                      Reassurance and follow-up of these patients and
                      families is necessary.

18.5 A **True**   The pathological process in asthma leads to
      B **True**   bronchospasm, mucosal oedema, and mucous
      C **False**   secretion. These changes are brought about by the
      D **False**   mediators which are released by the mast cells.
      E **True**   There are changes in the smooth muscle, alteration
                      in neural control and evidence of bronchial
                      inflammation leading to narrowing of the airways.
                      There are various factors such as viral infections,
                      allergens, seasonal variations and emotional stress
                      factors which could precipitate asthmatic attacks.

18.6 A **True**   The inflammation affects the bronchioles. The virus
      B **True**   colonizes the bronchiolar epithelium and replicates
      C **False**   there which leads to epithelial damage and necrosis.
      D **True**   The inflammatory cells infiltrate the bronchial walls.
      E **False**   There is oedema and congestion of the submucous
                      and adventitial tissue. The bronchiolar lumen
                      contains mucus, plugs of desquamated epithelial
                      cells and strands of fibrin. This could lead to
                      collapse of some of the alveoli with compensatory
                      hyperinflation of other alveoli. There is marked
                      increase of the functional residual capacity,
                      increased pulmonary resistance and decreased
                      dynamic compliance. The respiratory work is
                      markedly increased. There is impairment of gas
                      exchange. Hand to hand transfer is most common.

18.7 Problems often encountered in cystic fibrosis include:
 A renal failure
 B colonization with *Pseudomonas cepacia*
 C skin sepsis
 D haemoptysis
 E poor weight gain pattern despite adequate intake of pancreatic supplements

18.8 Bronchiectasis:
 A is a form of suppurative lung disease
 B may arise in infants who have had recurrent attacks of bronchiolitis
 C in the early stages may be easily diagnosed by plain chest X-ray
 D may be seen in children who have had severe pneumonia which resulted in destructive changes in the bronchial tree and lung parenchyma
 E may be associated with male infertility

18.9 The cystic fibrosis gene:
 A is located on chromosome 9
 B encodes an ion regulating protein
 C most commonly contains a mutation at amino acid position 508
 D may be diagnosed antenatally
 E mutations may be characterized by direct gene analysis

18.10 The following statements regarding mechanical ventilation in children are correct:
 A it may be necessary in children with severe asthma when there is a progressive rise in the $PaCO_2$
 B there are complications in 25% of cases
 C cardiovascular changes occur when the intrathoracic pressure is increased
 D long-term ventilation can have psychosocial effects, e.g. sleep disturbances, eating disorders, incontinence
 E profound malnutrition may occur in children who are ventilated for a long time

18.7	A	**False**	The management of cystic fibrosis is carried out on a multidisciplinary basis. It includes prevention of respiratory infection, regular physiotherapy, assessment of respiratory function at regular intervals looking for pathological organisms such as *Pseudomonas aeruginosa, Pseudomonas cepacia, Staphylococci aureus* and *Haemophilus influenzae*. Other viral organisms could also affect the respiratory tract and cause significant deterioration in patients' respiratory function. Assessment of their dietary requirement must be monitored very closely and the dietician must see them at regular intervals.
	B	**True**	
	C	**False**	
	D	**True**	
	E	**True**	

18.8	A	**True**	Bronchiectasis is a form of suppurative lung disease which may be widespread or focal. When the disease is widespread there may not be a predisposing cause but in focal problems it follows lung collapse, bronchial obstruction or parenchymal abnormality. There are three main ways in which the disorder arises: in recurring attacks of bronchiolitis in young infants; attacks of acute pneumonia; and following respiratory infection with lung collapse and subsequent bacterial infection. A chest X-ray is not a useful tool in the diagnosis of the disease in the early stages. In cystic fibrosis and in immotile cilia syndrome (where there may be a high incidence of bronchiectasis) there is a high incidence of male infertility.
	B	**True**	
	C	**False**	
	D	**True**	
	E	**True**	

18.9	A	**False**	The cystic fibrosis gene is located on the long arm of chromosome 7. It encodes a protein of 1,480 amino It is called cystic fibrosis transmembrane regulator gene, or CFTR. The commonest mutation that has been identified is ΔF 508, but more than 300 mutations have been noted. The gene affects the chloride ion across all the membranes. Antenatal diagnosis is possible by chorionic villus sampling.
	B	**True**	
	C	**True**	
	D	**True**	
	E	**True**	

18.10	A	**True**	Patient complications include air leaks, infection, aspiration, oxygen toxicity, cardiovascular effects and the syndrome of inappropriate ADH. Long-term complications include damage to the respiratory tract, nutritional status and psychosocial problems. Complications of ventilation occur in about 25% of ventilated children, although most are minor and can be treated easily. Many complications can be avoided with careful monitoring and anticipation.
	B	**True**	
	C	**True**	
	D	**True**	
	E	**True**	

18.11 Complications of asthma include:
- A pneumothorax and pneumomediastinum
- B segmental collapse
- C bronchiectasis
- D haemoptysis
- E lung cyst

18.12 The following are responsible for the pathological process in asthma:
- A monohydroxyeicosateiraenoic acid induces bronchospasm
- B histamine causes mucosal oedema
- C bradykinin causes mucous secretion
- D prostaglandins increase bronchospasm
- E platelets induce bronchospasm

18.13 The following statements regarding bronchial hyperreactivity are correct:
- A patients with bronchial hyperreactivity have symptoms of asthma
- B patients with mild disease have long-term stability despite bronchial hyperreactivity
- C it can be demonstrated by allergen challenge
- D it has diurnal variation in asthmatic children
- E it decreases with age in non-asthmatic children

18.11 A **True**   The complications of asthma include an acute life-
       B **True**   threatening asthmatic attack described as status
       C **False**   asthmaticus. Pneumothorax and pneumo-
       D **False**   mediastinum are often encountered in patients when
       E **False**   the response to treatment in an acute attack is
                        ineffective. Segmental lobe collapse or lung collapse
                        occurs when there is complete obstruction of the
                        moderate to medium sized bronchi with thick
                        mucous plugging. There are hardly ever
                        complications of haemoptysis or lung cyst in asthma,
                        but they may be seen if there is an underlying cause
                        for the asthma. However, localized airway
                        obstructions may occur as a result of thick mucosal
                        plugging.

18.12 A **False**   The pathological process in asthma is produced by
       B **True**   bronchospasm, mucosal oedema and increased
       C **False**   mucous secretion. Mediators such as histamine,
       D **True**   prostaglandins, leukotrienes, bradykinin, platelet
       E **True**   activating factor and monohydroxyeicosateiraenoic
                        acids are secreted by the mast cells. The correct
                        effects are:
                        histamine – bronchospasm, mucosal oedema
                        prostaglandin – bronchospasm, mucosal oedema
                        bradykinin – mucosal oedema, bronchospasm
                        platelet activating factor – mucosal oedema,
                        bronchospasm
                        monohydroxyeicosateiraenoic acid – increased
                        mucous secretion
                        Leukotrienes have an effect on all the mechanisms;
                        prostaglandin generating factor causes increased
                        mucous secretion and thromboxane causes
                        bronchospasm.

18.13 A **False**   Bronchial hyperreactivity is a characteristic feature
       B **True**   in asthmatic children. All asthmatic children
       C **True**   demonstrate bronchial hyperreactivity and there are
       D **True**   non-asthmatic subjects who have bronchial
       E **True**   hyperreactivity. Measurement of bronchial
                        hyperreactivity adds very little to the plan of
                        management of asthmatic patients. However,
                        understanding of it helps to clarify some aspects of
                        the aetiological process.

18.14 Children at greater risk of developing asthma include:
- A girls with a family history of atopic problems
- B boys who develop eczema in the first year of life
- C those whose parents smoke
- D infants who have had an episode of bronchiolitis
- E preterm infants

18.15 When inhaled steroids are used in the treatment of asthma:
- A early use improves symptoms
- B oral candidiasis is a recognized problem
- C high doses may be associated with significant risk of growth retardation
- D bronchial hyperreactivity is increased
- E dysphonia occurs due to the direct steroid effect on adductor muscle of the larynx

18.16 The following are recognized features of the pathology of asthma:
- A at post mortem the lungs are found to be large and do not deflate
- B bronchial ciliated cells appear normal
- C there is hypertrophy and hyperplasia of the bronchial smooth muscle
- D intraluminal bronchial secretion of mucus
- E lamina propria of the bronchial wall has normal blood vessels

18.14   A   **False**   There are a number of risk factors for the
        B   **True**   development of asthma. These vary between boys
        C   **True**   and girls. Family history, age of onset of atopic
        D   **True**   symptoms such as rhinitis and eczema, are
        E   **True**   important aspects to be considered in the diagnosis
                           and management of asthma. The various risk factors
                           have an additive effect in the development of
                           asthma. Feeding practices, domestic pets,
                           psychosocial factors may not be associated in the
                           development of asthma but they have a significant
                           effect in precipitating attacks in asthmatic patients.

18.15   A   **True**   The use of steroids in asthma has been recognized
        B   **True**   as a major advance in the treatment of the condition.
        C   **True**   Inhaled steroids should have high topical and low
        D   **False**   systemic activity in order to enhance clinical
        E   **True**   improvement and minimize the risk of adverse
                           events. The steroid used must be biotransformed to
                           an inactive metabolite as soon as it enters the
                           circulation. The inhaled steroids are inactivated in
                           the liver once they are absorbed into the circulation.
                           Rinsing the mouth, use of appropriate device and
                           proper technique decreases the amount swallowed.
                           Adrenal function is affected when large doses of
                           inhaled steroids are used. Growth and development
                           may be affected with long-term use of high dose
                           inhaled steroids.

18.16   A   **True**   Pathological features of the lungs in asthma have
        B   **False**   been obtained from patients dying during a severe
        C   **True**   attack. Bronchial biopsies taken for diagnostic
        D   **True**   purposes have provided additional histological
        E   **False**   information. The classical histological feature is the
                           presence of intraluminal secretions which comprises
                           of mucus, shed surface epithelium, eosinophils and
                           neutrophils. The lining epithelial cells of the
                           bronchial walls are markedly oedematous. Ciliated
                           cells are damaged and the goblet cells appear more
                           numerous. The basement membrane is thickened.
                           The lamina propria is oedematous with marked
                           dilation of the vessels and there is cellular infiltration
                           with eosinophils and neutrophils.

18.17 The following are true of croup:
- A diagnosis is made on clinical grounds
- B it is seen commonly in infants
- C drooling is a common sign
- D some children suffer recurrent episodes
- E dexamethasone is effective in some cases

18.18 The following statements apply in congenital pulmonary lymphangiectasis:
- A it presents late in infancy
- B it is seen in babies with hydrops
- C it has chest radiographic features similar to hyaline membrane disease
- D pneumothorax is a recognized complication
- E abnormal lymphatic drainage leads to pleural effusion

18.19 The following statements regarding nasal obstruction in infancy are correct:
- A infants are obligatory nasal breathers
- B choanal atresia is a feature of CHARGE syndrome
- C it may lead to obstructive apnoea
- D topical decongestants are best used indefinitely
- E feeding may be a major problem

18.20 The following statements about nitric oxide are correct:
- A the major part of the exhaled air originates from the nasal airways
- B it causes chronic lung injury
- C it is an inflammatory mediator
- D it is used in the treatment of persistent fetal circulation because of its vasodilator effect
- E the increased amount in the environment – from car exhaust, cigarette smoke and gas cookers – may contribute to increased incidence of asthma

18.17 A **True** Viral croup (acute laryngotracheobronchitis) is a
     B **False** common childhood respiratory infection
     C **False** characterized by inspiratory stridor, hoarse voice
     D **True** and barking cough. Some children have multiple
     E **True** episodes of this disorder. Croup has been
                 considered a self-limiting disease. However, in some
                 acute situations, where the airflow to the lungs is
                 affected, immediate medical or surgical intervention
                 may be necessary.

18.18 A **False** Congenital pulmonary lymphangiectasis is a rare
     B **True** disorder which presents as intractable respiratory
     C **False** distress from birth. The lungs show a diffuse dilation
     D **True** of the interlobular and subpleural lymphatics. The
     E **True** condition has been found in babies with hydrops.
                 Prognosis is poor. Vesicles are seen on the pleural
                 surface at autopsy. Pleural effusion is a common
                 finding.

18.19 A **True** Nasal obstruction in infancy is common and often
     B **True** distressing to parents. The obstruction is most often
     C **True** caused by non-specific rhinitis but in certain
     D **False** situations can pose management difficulties and
     E **True** lead to failure to thrive and rarely to life-threatening
                 events. Disorders which could cause nasal
                 obstructing are choanal atresia, nasal pyriform
                 aperture stenosis, birth trauma to the nasal cavity,
                 infection, allergic rhinitis, rhinitis medicamentosa,
                 upper airway obstruction, craniofacial anomalies and
                 midline nasal masses.

18.20 A **True** Nitric oxide is an endothelium derived relaxing
     B **True** factor. It is involved in many biological processes. In
     C **True** the lungs it has a vasodilator, bronchodilator,
     D **True** neurotransmitter and inflammatory mediator
     E **True** function. It is produced in the endothelial cells by
                 enzymatic mechanism (nitric oxide synthase). As the
                 biological action is discovered it is being used in the
                 treatment of some clinical disorders.

18.21 Features of laryngomalacia include:
A spontaneous resolution of the symptoms during the second year
B increased resistance to flow of air during inspiration
C exacerbation of the symptoms during respiratory infections
D abnormal flow volume loops in older children
E absence in skeletal dysplasias

18.22 Bronchoscopy in children:
A is mainly used for diagnostic purposes
B requires a rigid bronchoscope for diagnostic purposes
C is contraindicated in severe hypoxaemia
D is indicated when there is poor response to treatment despite the use of bronchodilators, aggressive physiotherapy and antibiotics
E necessitates a rigid bronchoscope for the diagnosis of vocal cord dysfunction

18.23 The following statements about *Mycoplasma* pneumonia are correct:
A it occurs commonly in infancy
B symptoms are worse than the signs elicited by auscultation of the chest
C sickle cell disease patients suffer a mild infection
D localized areas of bronchospasm is a diagnostic feature
E co-trimoxazole is the treatment of choice

18.24 The following statements apply in recurrent inhalation:
A failure to thrive may occur
B upper gastrointestinal anatomical abnormalities may predispose to the illness
C pH studies may be essential to make a definite diagnosis of gastro-oesophageal reflux
D it occurs in the CHARGE syndrome
E bronchodilator therapy may help to relieve some of the chest symptoms

18.21	A	**True**	Laryngomalacia is characterized by inspiratory stridor beginning at birth or soon after it, which is exacerbated by crying and respiratory infections. In some instances there may be feeding problems. The condition may be associated with skeletal dysplasias. Body plethysmography has shown an increase in both inspiratory and expiratory resistance. The symptoms may last more than 2 years. These patients may require closer supervision because the airflow may become affected during respiratory illnesses.
	B	**True**	
	C	**True**	
	D	**True**	
	E	**False**	

18.22	A	**False**	The development of rigid and flexible bronchoscopes has been useful for diagnostic purposes as well as for therapeutic purposes. The flexible bronchoscope helps to study the mean dynamic airway function. This procedure is carried out under sedation. The rigid bronchoscope requires general anaesthesia and is reserved mainly for therapeutic procedures such as removal of foreign bodies or large amounts of material from the airways.
	B	**False**	
	C	**True**	
	D	**True**	
	E	**True**	

18.23	A	**False**	*Mycoplasma* pneumonia is a common cause of pneumonia in schoolchildren and young adults; it rarely affects infants. The symptoms are often worse than the signs and those with sickle cell disease, congenital heart disease or chronic lung problems are severely affected. The drug of choice is erythromycin or a newer macrolide.
	B	**True**	
	C	**False**	
	D	**False**	
	E	**False**	

18.24	A	**True**	Recurrent inhalation is an underdiagnosed clinical problem; it can often present with failure to thrive and is also seen in upper gastrointestinal anatomical abnormalities such as cleft palate, macroglossia and laryngeal cleft. pH studies have been helpful in the diagnosis of gastro-oesophageal reflux. Recurrent inhalation problems also are seen in CHARGE syndrome, which includes coloboma of the eyes, hare lip, cardiac defect, rib abnormalities and gastro-oesophageal reflux. Bronchodilators may be helpful to relieve bronchospasm which occurs often in recurrent inhalation problems.
	B	**True**	
	C	**True**	
	D	**True**	
	E	**True**	

18.25 Correct statements regarding lung growth disorders include:
  A they develop when there is decreased intrathoracic lung space
  B reduction of fetal lung movements may occur in maternal diabetes mellitus
  C antenatal ultrasound may be useful in detecting pleural effusion
  D renal tract anomalies are associated with poor lung growth
  E the prognosis is poor in small chest syndrome

18.26 Wheezing in infancy is associated with:
  A diaphragmatic hernia
  B vascular rings
  C cystic fibrosis
  D asthma
  E *Mycoplasma pneumoniae* infection

18.27 The following are true of miliary tuberculosis:
  A it affects two or more organs
  B it is commonest in infants and young children
  C lymphadenopathy and hepatomegaly are recognized features in the early stages
  D it may present as 'pyrexia of unknown origin'
  E chest X-ray abnormalities resolve soon after commencing treatment

18.28 In tuberculous meningitis:
  A symptoms are non-specific, e.g. fever, malaise, irritability, drowsiness
  B convulsions occur in the late stages
  C cerebrospinal fluid protein is very high
  D all patients have a positive tuberculin test
  E hydrocephalus is a recognized complication

18.25 A **True**   Many factors could affect the lung growth during the
B **False**   intrauterine period. They could occur as a result of
C **True**   intrathoracic compressions such as in diaphragmatic
D **True**   hernia, diminished fetal lung breathing activity such
E **True**   as in muscle disorders, and decreased production of amniotic fluid as in Potter's syndrome. Antenatal ultrasound may be useful in the detection of some congenital anomalies.

18.26 A **False**   Wheezing in infancy may occur in obstructive
B **False**   disease of the small airways or in obstructive lesions
C **True**   of the trachea or the major bronchi. In the former it
D **True**   may be acute, recurrent or persistent. The most
E **False**   common acute disease that causes wheezing is acute viral bronchiolitis.

18.27 A **True**   Miliary tuberculosis is an early complication of
B **True**   primary infection. Numerous tubercle bacilli are
C **False**   released from the primary focus into the blood
D **True**   stream; they lodge in the smaller capillaries in
E **False**   different organs. Miliary tuberculosis is more common in infants, malnourished children, and immune suppressed patients. The patient becomes gravely ill over several days. 30% of these patients have a negative Mantoux test. Biopcy of the liver or bone marrow may facilitate rapid diagnosis. Resolution is slow even with correct treatment.

18.28 A **True**   Tuberculous meningitis is a serious complication. It
B **True**   occurs as a result of the formation of a metastatic
C **True**   caseous lesion on the cortex or the meninges. Onset
D **False**   of the symptoms may be insidious or abrupt. The
E **True**   disease is rare in infants under 4 months of age. The progression of the disease is usually in three stages: in the first the symptoms are mainly non-specific; in the second obvious neurological symptoms develop, e.g. convulsions, lethargy, abnormal clinical signs; and in the third there is coma, irregular pulse and respiration, hypertension, decerebate posturing and eventually death.

18.29 The following antituberculous drugs used in children have these adverse effects:
- A streptomycin – hepatotoxicity
- B rifampicin – staining of contact lenses
- C pyrazinamide – arthritis and arthralgia
- D ethambutol – eye damage
- E capreomycin – kidney damage

18.29 A **False** A variety of antituberculous drugs are used in
     B **True**   children and all of them have adverse effects. Due to
     C **True**   the emergence of drug resistance the choice of drug
     D **True**   would depend on epidemiologic factors, resistance
     E **True**   of the organism and the clinical state of the patient.
                  The usual principle of antituberculous drug therapy
                  is the use of a bactericidal drug, along with a second
                  drug to prevent the emergence of a resistant strain.
                  In certain countries triple or quadruple therapy is
                  used. The first line drugs include isoniazid,
                  rifampicin, ethambutol and streptomycin. The
                  second line drugs include para-aminosalicylic acid,
                  ethionamide, capreomycin, kanamycin and
                  cycloserine.

19. Embryology

19.1 In the development of the heart:
- **A** the lateral endocardial tubes in the cardiogenic region of the embryo fuse to form the primitive heart tube
- **B** the primitive ventricle folds and separates to form the right and left ventricle
- **C** the cardiac jelly forms the myocardial muscle
- **D** the atrioventricular valves are formed from the ventricular myocardium
- **E** the contruncus develops into the distal outflow regions of the right and the left ventricles

19.2 The following statements about the fetomaternal circulation are correct:
- **A** uteroplacental circulation develops in the third week after fertilization
- **B** the placenta contains approximately 150 ml of maternal blood and this volume is replaced about 3 or 4 times per minute
- **C** the antibodies that cross the placenta into the fetus disappear in the neonate in the first month
- **D** the placenta produces steroid hormones and prostaglandins
- **E** carbon dioxide, urea and uric acid pass from the maternal circulation into the fetal blood

19.1　A　**True**　　The cardiogenic region is recognizable as a
　　　B　**False**　　flattened structure around the fifteenth day after
　　　C　**False**　　fertilization. In this region the angioblastic cords
　　　D　**True**　　coalesce to form a pair of lateral endocardial tubes.
　　　E　**True**　　The cephalic and lateral folding of the embryo during the fourth week causes the tubes to be brought together along the midline to fuse to form the primitive heart tube. Thereafter the process of folding, remodelling and septation leads to the embryonic stage of the four-chambered heart. Further differentiation of the tissues of the embryonic heart progresses through gestation (and to an identifiable fetal heart around 23 weeks' gestation).

19.2　A　**True**　　The embryo derives the nutrients and eliminates the
　　　B　**True**　　wastes by a simple process of diffusion in the first
　　　C　**False**　　week. As it grows, the process of transfer of material
　　　D　**True**　　becomes more complex and there is a need for the
　　　E　**False**　　development of the uteroplacental circulation. The trophoblastic lacunae start developing around the ninth day within the syncytiotrophoblast. The maternal capillaries in this area expand to form the maternal sinusoids. The proliferation of the cytotrophoblast and the formation of the processes result in the primary stem villi. The extension and the growth of the extraembryonic mesoderm into the primary stem villi gives rise to the secondary stem villi. Further differentiation of the mesoderm forms the blood vessels which subsequently connect with the vessels forming in the embryo. This differentiated structure is called tertiary stem villi. The gases, nutrients and wastes that diffuse between the maternal and fetal blood pass four layers, viz. the endothelium of the villus capillaries, villus connective tissue, a layer of cytotrophoblast and a layer of syncytiotrophoblast.

19.3 **The following events occur during gametogenesis and fertilization:**
A spermatogenesis begins in fetal life
B oogenesis begins in the fetal ovary
C embryonic membranes develop during gastrulation
D in organogenesis the differentiation of the central nervous system occurs first
E the blastocyst is formed in the ampulla of the oviduct

19.4 **The following statements regarding lung growth and development are correct:**
A the canalicular stage of development is in the first week after birth
B the lung develops from the primitive foregut as a ventral diverticulum
C budding and branching of the lung bud continues up to the sixteenth week of gestation
D surfactant storage in the alveolar type II epithelial cells occurs during the pseudoglandular stage
E alveoli are fully developed in the full-term infant

19.5 **In cardiogenesis**
A the primitive heart tube folds to the left in dextrocardia
B the superior and inferior endocardial cushions fail to fuse in atrioventricular septal defects
C the right ventricle is hypoplastic in double-outlet left ventricle
D the truncoconal septa fails to develop in transposition of the great vessels
E the truncoconal septa is well differentiated in persistent truncus arteriosus

19.3 A **False**   There are five stages in the development of the
     B **True**   fetus. In fertilization the gametes fuse in the ampulla
     C **True**   of the oviduct. The fused structure (zygote) travels
     D **True**   down the oviduct, during which stage there is
     E **False**   division of the cells (cleavage). The cells form a
                   spherical mass (morula). It in turn develops into a
                   fluid-filled mass of cells (blastocyst). The blastocyst
                   hatches out to implant onto the prepared
                   endometrium of the uterine wall. In gastrulation the
                   extraembryonic membranes form and the inner cell
                   mass becomes a flat sheet, which lies between the
                   amniotic cavity and the yolk sac. In organogenesis
                   the cells of the embryo undergo further
                   differentiation and morphogenesis to form the
                   specific tissues and organs.

19.4 A **False**   The lungs begin to develop in the fourth week and
     B **True**   begin to mature just before birth. There are four
     C **True**   stages of fetal lung development: embryonic
     D **False**   pseudoglandular, canalicular and terminal sac. The
     E **False**   lung bud is recognized as a diverticulum of the
                   primitive foregut around the fourth week of gestation.
                   The branching of the lung bud in the following days
                   produces the two lungs, the lung lobes and the
                   bronchopulmonary segments. During the
                   pseudoglandular stage, from 6 to 16 weeks,
                   generations of branching results in the formation of
                   terminal bronchioles. The respiratory vasculature
                   develops during the canalicular stage and the
                   terminal bronchioles subdivide to form the
                   respiratory bronchioles. Alveoli develop from the
                   saccules during the terminal development stage.
                   The terminal sacs continue to be produced until
                   well into childhood.

19.5 A **False**   Cardiovascular malformation is the most common
     B **True**   type of life-threatening congenital defect in the
     C **True**   neonatal period. Several factors could affect the
     D **True**   development of the heart, e.g. chromosomal
     E **False**   anomalies, intrauterine infections. Any variation in
                   the normal process of the development may result in
                   a malformation. The type of defect depends on the
                   stage at which the development of the heart was
                   affected. Neural crest migration, haemodynamic
                   forces and programmed cell death are factors which
                   play an essential role in the pathogenesis of
                   congenital heart disease.

19.6 The following statements are true of the development of the gastrointestinal tract:
  A the gut in the embryo is distinguishable in the fourth week as a double-ended blind tube
  B the spleen is derived from the gut tube endoderm
  C the mesodermal coating of the gut tube gives rise to the submucosal connective tissue and the smooth muscle layer
  D the primary intestinal loop herniates into the umbilicus in the sixth week
  E Meckel's diverticulum is an anomaly of the vitelline duct

19.7 Which of the following statements relating to the development of the genital system are correct:
  A the primordial germ cells migrate from the yolk sac
  B male and female sex differentiation is recognizable by the end of the fifth week
  C sex determining region of the Y chromosomes influences the production of the testis determining factor in the sex cord cells
  D the urethral fold gives rise to the vestibule of the vagina
  E the testis and the ovaries both develop in the region of the 10th thoracic level

19.8 The following statements apply in the development of the eyes:
  A the optic primordia are identifiable in the region of the forebrain in the third week
  B the lens is formed from the tissue of the optic vesicle
  C the hyaloid branch of the ophthalmic artery vascularizes the retina
  D the inner wall of the optic cup gives rise to the neural retina
  E the iris and the ciliary body are formed from the rim of the optic cup and the choroidal mesenchyme

19.6 A **True**   The gut tube is differentiated in the embryo to the
      B **False**   foregut, midgut and hindgut. From this arises the
      C **True**   different regions of the gut from the pharynx to the
      D **True**   rectum. Also from the foregut develop the
      E **True**   pharyngeal pouch and its derivatives, lungs, liver
                        and its appendages, pancreas, and urogenital sinus
                        and its derivatives. The endodermal folding of the
                        embryo commences in the fourth week and the
                        differentiation continues until the twelfth week. The
                        primitive tube elongates and subsequently rotates in
                        the proximal part then loops in the area of the
                        midgut and later rotates. Disturbance of
                        developments during this stage results in a variety of
                        clinical disorders including incomplete canalization,
                        anterior abdominal wall defects as well as
                        malrotation of the gut.

19.7 A **True**   The development of the genital system begins
      B **False**   around the sixth week when the germ cells migrate
      C **True**   from the yolk sac. Around this time the cells
      D **False**   adjoining the mesonephros and the coelomic
      E **True**   epithelium differentiate into somatic sex cord cells,
                        as the sex cords differentiate into the Sertoli cells in
                        males and follicular cells in females. Differentiation
                        of the sex cord cells is determined by the encoding
                        gene on the Y chromosome. Further maturation and
                        the development of the Sertoli cells influence the
                        development of the male genitalia. In females the
                        mesenchymal cells supporting the sex cords
                        differentiate into follicles and the genital ridge
                        becomes the ovary. The external genitalia develop
                        from the pair of labioscrotal folds, pair of urogenital
                        folds and anterior tubercle.

19.8 A **True**   The eyes develop from the forebrain in the fourth
      B **False**   week. The optic sulci develops into optic vesicles,
      C **True**   optic cup and the optic stalk. These structures give
      D **True**   rise to the retina and the optic nerve. The lens
      E **True**   develop from an ectodermal placode that forms
                        adjacent to the optic cup. The nerve fibres from the
                        retina grow through the optic stalk and transform it
                        into the optic nerve. The mesenchymal capsule of
                        the optic vesicle gives rise to the choroid, the sclera
                        and the anterior chamber. The rim of the optic cup
                        and the overlying mesenchyme form the iris and the
                        ciliary body. The extrinsic ocular muscles develop
                        from the mesenchyme adjacent to the optic cup. The
                        surface ectoderm and associated mesenchyme
                        develop into the iris.

19.9 The following statements apply in the development of the integumentary system:
A the dermis is a mesodermal tissue
B the ectoderm differentiates into the periderm and basal layer after neurulation
C the hair follicles arise from the periderm
D the secondary tooth buds arise independently from the dental lamina
E the mammary glands are modified apocrine glands

19.10 The following changes occur in the development of the pituitary gland:
A it develops entirely from the infundibulum of the third ventricle
B cells of the infundibulum differentiate into the pars intermedia and neurohypophysis
C craniopharyngiomas are tumours of the Rathke's pouch
D the diencephalic pouch develops in the second trimester
E the lumen of the diencephalic infundibulum persists throughout the intrauterine period

19.11 In the development of the kidneys:
A kidney architecture is created between the fifth and fifteenth week of gestation
B the nephrons are developed from the ureteric bud
C the metanephric blastema develops from the intermediate mesoderm on each side of the body axis
D the cervical nephrotomes function as fetal kidneys
E the bladder develops from the anterior primitive urogenital sinus

19.9	A	**True**	The integumentary system consists of the skin, hair, epidermal glands, nails and teeth. The skin consists of the epidermis and the dermis. The epidermis is primarily formed from the embryonic surface ectoderm, which further differentiates into periderm and basal layer after neurulation. The basal layer gives rise to the intermediate layer and the stratum germinativum. The latter gives rise to three further layers which contain keratinocytes. The dermis contains structures of the skin such as blood vessels, nerves, muscle bundles and sensory structures. The skin gives rise to specialized structures such as hair, nails and epidermal glands.
	B	**True**	
	C	**False**	
	D	**False**	
	E	**True**	
19.10	A	**False**	The ventral outpouching of the diencephalic floor plate is the infundibulum, which gives rise to the posterior pituitary. The Rathke's pouch, which arises from the stomadeal roof, gives rise to the anterior pituitary. This differentiation is seen in the third week.
	B	**True**	
	C	**True**	
	D	**False**	
	E	**False**	
19.11	A	**True**	The intermediate mesoderm on either side of the axial line give rise to the nephric structures developing from the cervical area (nephrotome), followed by the mesonephri in the thoracic and lumbar area, and finally the metanephri in the sacral area – the definitive kidneys. The nephric development starts in the fourth week of gestation. The ureters and the collecting duct systems develop from the ureteric buds, whilst the nephrons are differentiated from the metanephric blastema. The kidneys ascend from the original region to the lumbar site. The bladder and the urethra develop from the anterior segment of the urogenital sinus.
	B	**False**	
	C	**True**	
	D	**False**	
	E	**True**	

20. Nephrology

20.1 The following statements regarding the investigation of a child with haematuria are correct:
    A the tests performed depend on the information obtained from the history, examination and urinalysis
    B urine culture is essential if haematuria is confirmed
    C renal biopsy is recommended when persistent mild proteinuria is also present
    D a hearing test is indicated when familial nephritis is suspected
    E ultrasound of the renal tract detects small areas of calcification

20.2 In systemic lupus erythematosus:
    A more males are affected than females
    B arthritis and dermatitis occur in the early stages
    C a falling concentration of serum C4 is a reliable indicator of disease activity
    D the histology of the kidneys is variable
    E an assay of anti-double-stranded DNA antibodies is critical for evaluating disease activity

20.3 Hypernatraemia may:
    A be countered in child abuse
    B be seen occasionally in sickle cell disease
    C occur in formula-fed infants
    D cause a high urinary sodium excretion in hypernatraemic dehydration
    E occur in premature infants placed under radiant warmers

20.1 A **True**   Haematuria may be a presenting feature when it is
      B **True**   gross. A detailed history, careful clinical examination
      C **False**   and urine analysis help to plan the investigations.
      D **True**   The causes of haematuria include infection,
      E **False**   glomerular diseases, renal calculi, trauma,
                     anatomical abnormalities, vascular (e.g. arteritis,
                     infarction, thrombosis), haematological and exercise
                     induced. The investigations would depend on the
                     suspected cause. Investigations include urine
                     culture, haematological and biochemical tests,
                     radiological examination, tests for
                     glomerulonephritis, hearing tests and renal biopsy.

20.2 A **False**   Systemic lupus erythematosus is a multisystem
      B **True**   disease in which widespread inflammation of the
      C **True**   connective tissues and immune complex vasculitis
      D **True**   occur. Immunological, environmental and hereditary
      E **True**   factors have been implicated in the cause of the
                     disease. It is uncommon in children under 5 years of
                     age but becomes more common during
                     adolescence. There are varying clinical
                     manifestations either at the onset or during the
                     course of the disease. There are specific indications
                     for the use of steroids and other immunosuppressive
                     drugs.

20.3 A **True**   Hypernatraemia may arise from inadequate water
      B **True**   intake, excessive sodium intake or disproportionate
      C **True**   loss of water to sodium. The common cause of
      D **False**   excessive water loss is nephrogenic diabetes
      E **True**   insipidus, which may be inherited, or following renal
                     insults due to drugs or kidney disease.
                     Hypernatraemic dehydration is relatively uncommon
                     in children following diarrhoea and vomiting. The
                     problem is well recognized in overenthusiastic use of
                     formula milk in infants. These infants may present
                     with neurological symptoms.

20.4 The following statements about Wilms tumour are true:
A it is an embryonic tumour
B increased secretion of glycosaminoglycans may cause life-threatening hyperviscosity syndrome
C its staging is essential at the time of diagnosis to assess the prognosis
D it is not sensitive to radiotherapy
E chest radiography may show metastatic nodules

20.5 In renal stone disease:
A *Proteus mirabilis*, an infective agent, precipitates renal stones
B mucopolysaccharides, citrates and pyrophosphates inhibit the growth of renal stones
C adenine phosphoribosyl transferase deficiency causes renal stones which are not easily crushable
D idiopathic hypercalciuria is an autosomal recessive disorder
E treatment of cystinuria with D-penicillamine precipitates proteinuria

20.6 Renal tubular acidosis:
A type I is caused by a defect in bicarbonate reabsorption
B the proximal form is due to an impaired sodium/hydrogen ion exchange mechanism
C the proximal form may be transient in infants and neonates
D type IV is associated with hyperchloraemia and hyperkalaemia
E type II is a recognized side-effect of amphotericin B therapy

20.4 A **True**   Wilms tumour is a malignant embryonal neoplasm of
     B **True**   mixed histology. It is extremely sensitive to
     C **True**   chemotherapeutic agents and radiation. Patients
     D **False**   often present with abdominal distension, noted by
     E **True**   health visitors, parents or relatives. There may be no
                    systemic upset. Some patients have hypertension
                    which is mostly renovascular in origin. The other
                    causes of hypertension must be excluded prior to
                    surgery because of anaesthetic and surgical risks.
                    Histology and staging of the Wilms tumour, based on
                    the US National Wilms Tumour Study (NWTS) and
                    the UKCCSG studies, are essential for management
                    and to assess prognosis.

20.5 A **True**   Renal stones are rare in children. They may be
     B **True**   identified when the child presents with
     C **False**   gastrointestinal symptoms. They may be infective,
     D **True**   hypercalcaemic (absorptive or renal type) or
     E **True**   metabolic (cystinuria, oxalate, purine) and may also
                    be seen in tumour lysis syndrome. Drugs may
                    precipitate renal stones (corticosteroid excess).
                    Affected children present with abdominal pain,
                    haematuria or urinary tract infections. Careful history
                    taking is essential in order to exclude a familial
                    cause.

20.6 A **False**   Renal tubular acidosis (RTA) is a biochemical
     B **True**   syndrome characterized by persistent
     C **True**   hyperchloraemic metabolic acidosis and
     D **True**   abnormalities in the renal regulation of bicarbonate
     E **True**   concentration. At least four types have been
                    described. The classical distal RTA (type I) is a
                    Mendelian dominant characteristic, but it may also
                    be secondary to systemic lupus erythematosus,
                    sickle cell disease, and renal disease such as
                    pyelonephritis. In the proximal RTA (type II) there is
                    a defect of bicarbonate reabsorption. This disorder
                    can be primary or secondary in association with
                    Fanconi syndrome. Toxins such as lead could give
                    rise to type II RTA.

20.7 **The following statements apply to proteinuria:**
A a pathological aetiology is strenuous exercise
B it is seen in up to 3% of school children
C urine protein excretion of more than 40 mg/m^2 is associated with hypoalbuminuria
D it occurs in 40–50% of children with IgA nephropathy
E Tamm-Horsfall protein is not found in normal urine

20.8 **The following statements regarding glomerulonephritis in children are correct:**
A it is an immune mechanism which affects the structure and function of both kidneys
B D-penicillamine induces immune complex mechanisms causing glomerular damage
C presentation may be with asymptomatic haematuria or proteinuria
D hypertension is not a recognized feature in acute post-streptococcal glomerulonephritis
E Henoch-Schönlein purpura nephritis affects children between 3 and 10 years of age

20.9 **The following statements about rapidly progressive glomerulonephritis are correct:**
A crescent formation is the most commonly associated histological feature
B anaemia is rare
C it is recognized in Goodpasture's syndrome
D it is seen in bacterial endocarditis
E hypertension, haematuria and oedema are early features

20.7 A False
     B True
     C True
     D True
     E False

Urinary protein measurement is an investigation in the diagnosis and management of renal disease. In disorders such as familial nephrolithiasis, uncomplicated obstructive uropathy and interstitial nephritis, proteinuria does not increase with the progress of the disease. Proteinuria is measured by the dipstick method or by quantitative tests. Qualitative assessment is used in the diagnosis of glomerular and tubular disorders.

20.8 A True
     B True
     C True
     D False
     E True

Glomerulonephritis is a result of an immune process that damages the structure and the functioning of the glomeruli. The pathogenesis has been extensively studied, and injury has been attributed to immune complexes, coagulation factors and exogenous toxins. The clinical presentations are acute nephritic syndrome, chronic glomerulonephritis, rapidly progressive glomerulonephritis and nephrotic syndrome. A clear history and detailed examination are necessary to plan the laboratory investigations. These include urine analysis, both microscopically and chemically, as well as renal function and immunological tests.

20.9 A True
     B False
     C True
     D True
     E True

Rapidly progressive glomerulonephritis clinically shows rapid deterioration in renal function from uraemia to end stage renal failure. This disorder may be primary or secondary in association with infection or other systemic disease. Histologically, crescent formation is often seen, and the rapid enlargement of the crescent damages the glomerular function. Therapy is aimed at stopping glomerular injury. High-dose steroids and cytotoxic drugs have been used in therapy. Supportive therapy in associated disorders is essential. End stage renal disease requires renal dialysis or renal transplant.

20.10 Features of prune-belly syndrome include:
  A respiratory illness in the neonatal period
  B restrictive lung disease as a complication in childhood
  C renal tract anomalies not associated with this condition
  D end stage renal failure developing in the third or fourth week
  E constipation

20.11 The following investigations are appropriate in a girl of 8 months following her first proven uncomplicated urinary tract infection:
  A renal ultrasound
  B plain abdominal X-ray
  C intravenous urogram
  D DMSA renal static scan
  E DTPA dynamic indirect cystogram

20.12 The following are recognized causes of hypertension:
  A patent ductus arteriosus
  B renal artery stenosis
  C multiple scarred kidney
  D phaeochromocytoma
  E steroid therapy

20.13 Recognized causes of neonatal renal vein thrombosis include:
  A perinatal asphyxia
  B polycythaemia
  C hypernatraemia
  D hypoglycaemia
  E twin-twin transfusion

20.14 Complications of nephrotic syndrome include:
  A spontaneous bacterial peritonitis
  B abdominal pain
  C hypertensive crisis
  D thrombosis
  E acute renal failure

20.10	A	True	Prune-belly syndrome (the Eagle-Barrett syndrome) is a congenital disorder that classically consists of deficient abdominal musculature, urinary tract abnormality, renal hypoplasia or dysplasia, and cryptorchidism. Pulmonary and renal dysfunction predominate. Pulmonary hypoplasia secondary to oligohydramnios can result in varying degrees of respiratory insufficiency in the newborn. During childhood respiratory illness is common. The urinary tract findings are similar to those of posterior urethral valves with the exception of an obstruction. Hence monitoring of the urinary output and renal function is part of the management. Replacement of salt, correcting metabolic acidosis and providing an activated form of vitamin D are included in the management.
	B	True	
	C	False	
	D	False	
	E	True	
20.11	A	True	Guidelines for investigation of urinary tract infections vary widely. Most agree that an ultrasound is mandatory. Many suggest a DMSA scan to ensure that there is no evidence of minor renal scarring plus an estimate of renal differential function. An intravenous urogram is not routine. A plain X-ray is usually of benefit for the location of calculi if these are suspected clinically. This child is too young for an indirect DTPA cystogram and therefore would warrant a micturating cystourethrogram.
	B	False	
	C	False	
	D	True	
	E	False	
20.12	A	False	Renal disease is the most common cause of hypertension. Coarctation of the aorta rather than patent ductus arteriosus is the cardiac aetiology.
	B	True	
	C	True	
	D	True	
	E	True	
20.13	A	True	Renal vein thrombosis occurs in the presence of haemoconcentration, dehydration or polycythaemia.
	B	True	
	C	True	
	D	False	
	E	True	
20.14	A	True	All are well-recognized complications of nephrotic syndrome. Abdominal pain and hypertension are features of hypovolaemia.
	B	True	
	C	True	
	D	True	
	E	True	

20.15 **Indications of severe hypovolaemia during the polyuric treatment phase of nephrotic syndrome include:**
- A colloid dependent abdominal pain
- B capillary refill time of 3 seconds
- C urinary specific gravity of 1040
- D core-periphery temperature gap of 20
- E hypotension

20.15 A **True**   Hypovolaemia is a serious complication encountered
       B **False**   during the polyuric phase of nephrotic syndrome.
       C **True**   Abdominal pain may respond to colloid infusion. An
       D **True**   increasing urinary specific gravity suggests
       E **True**   dehydration/hypovolaemia. A capillary refill time of
                       2–3 seconds is normal.

21. Liver and gastroenterology

21.1 In Wilson's disease:
- A the prevalence worldwide is about 1 per 50 000
- B serum caeruloplasmin may be normal
- C lung involvement is an early feature
- D early liver biopsy shows characteristic rubaenic staining for rubaenic acid
- E deteriorating behaviour is a non-hepatic clinical presentation

21.2 Features of extrahepatic biliary atresia include:
- A jaundice developing at 3–6 weeks of age
- B acholic stools
- C associated defects such as polysplenia
- D conjugated hyperbilirubinaemia
- E imaging using imidodiacetic acid derivatives helps to differentiate from neonatal hepatitis

21.3 The following statements regarding gastro-oesophageal reflux are correct:
- A it is seen in mentally retarded children with or without hiatus hernia
- B it is associated with apparent life-threatening events
- C diagnosis should be considered in babies with persistent bronchospasm
- D it presents as choking during feeds
- E when not associated with other disorders the symptoms improve with complete functional maturity in 60–70% of the patients

21.1 A **True**   Wilson's disease is an inborn error of copper
      B **True**   metabolism. Accumulation of toxic amounts of
      C **False**   copper in liver, brain, kidney and cornea leads to
      D **False**   both hepatic and non-hepatic clinical presentation. It
      E **True**   has an estimated worldwide prevalence of 1 per
                     50 000. 23% of children with Wilson's disease have
                     normal serum caeruloplasmin. Rubaenic acid
                     staining is characteristically positive at the late
                     stages of the disease. Without treatment there is
                     progressive damage to the liver and brain, and
                     premature death.

21.2 A **True**   Extrahepatic biliary atresia is amenable to surgical
      B **True**   treatment. There is hypoplasia or atresia of any
      C **True**   portion of the extrahepatic system. The clinical
      D **True**   condition is easily mistaken for neonatal hepatitis.
      E **True**   The aetiology of the atresia is unknown. Viral and
                     genetic insults during organogenesis have been
                     postulated. Systematic investigations to identify
                     known causes of neonatal hepatitis are required.
                     Treatment is surgery, and the best results are
                     obtained when surgery is carried out by 60 days of
                     age.

21.3 A **True**   Gastro-oesophageal reflux is easily and well
      B **True**   controlled. In most children the symptoms resolve by
      C **True**   18–20 months of age when not associated with
      D **False**   other disorders. In this condition there is retrograde
      E **True**   movement of the contents of the stomach into the
                     oesophagus. This may occur in structural anomalies,
                     chromosomal anomalies, neurological and muscular
                     disorders. The availability of pH monitoring in the
                     oesophagus and the use of prokinetic agents have
                     improved the management of this condition.

21.4 **The following statements apply in pancreatic enzyme insufficiency:**
  A cystic fibrosis is the commonest associated disorder
  B secretin-pancreozymin is the most direct test for assessing pancreatic function
  C paucity of interlobular bile ducts is associated with partial exocrine pancreatic insufficiency
  D growth delay, skeletal dysplasia and neutropenia are not associated with this disorder
  E immune reactive trypsin levels progressively increase with the destruction of the pancreas

21.5 **In recurrent abdominal pain in childhood:**
  A the periumbilical is the commonest site described by children
  B gastro-oesophageal reflux is a recognized cause
  C children under 5 years of age complaining of abdominal pain are colonized by *Helicobacter pylori* in the gastric antrum
  D urine microbiology is an essential part of the medical assessment
  E taste-induced phobia is a recognized problem

21.6 **The following statements regarding Crohn's disease are correct:**
  A it affects continuous segment of the bowel
  B excessive intake of carbohydrate has been incriminated in the pathogenesis of the disease
  C pyoderma gangrenosum is a recognized feature
  D arthritis is common in colonic involvement
  E it affects any segment of the gastrointestinal tract

21.4 A **True**   Pancreatic insufficiency is a well-recognized
      B **True**   problem in cystic fibrosis, the Schwachman-
      C **True**   Diamond syndrome, congenital pancreatic
      D **False**   hypoplasia and in malnutrition. These children
      E **False**   present with features of malabsorption. Partial
                     pancreatic insufficiency has been described in
                     association with paucity of the interlobular bile ducts.
                     The direct evaluation of pancreatic function is by
                     stimulation of the pancreas by the hormones,
                     secretin and pancreozymin. The indirect tests
                     include 72 hour faecal fat analysis, stool trypsin and
                     chymotrypsin, and measurement of immune reactive
                     trypsin. The other indirect test, not invasive, is the
                     measurement of urinary or plasma para-
                     aminobenzoic acid following the oral administration
                     of synthetic chymotrypsin substrate containing para-
                     aminobenzoic acid.

21.5 A **True**   Recurrent abdominal pain in childhood is a common
      B **True**   problem. Careful medical assessment is essential to
      C **False**   exclude an organic cause. The symptom often
      D **True**   affects at least 10% of the children over 5 years of
      E **True**   age. Most studies have encouraged a conservative
                     approach to investigations if the abdominal pain was
                     the only symptom with no clinical finding. The family
                     history and the psychological assessment is
                     essential in order to plan the appropriate course of
                     action.

21.6 A **False**   The clinical presentation of Crohn's disease
      B **True**   depends on the site of the lesion and the extent of
      C **True**   the inflammatory lesion. The features include the
      D **True**   symptoms of extraintestinal involvement and growth
      E **True**   involvement, small bowel symptoms and colonic
                     features. Poor growth and under-nutrition occurs in
                     the majority of the children during the course of the
                     illness. The complications in the gut occur due to the
                     transmural involvement of the gut wall. Skin tags,
                     anal fissures, perianal or perirectal abscesses may
                     arise during the onset of the disease or during
                     exacerbation of the disease process. Diagnosis of
                     the disease is made on the clinical features,
                     radiological appearance of the gut wall and
                     histology. The aim of therapy includes to minimize
                     the exacerbation of the disease process.
                     Pharmacological and nutritional therapy is essential
                     immediately after diagnosis. Surgery is reserved for
                     acute and chronic complications of the disease.

21.7 **The following are true of rotavirus diarrhoea:**
    A it is caused by a reovirus
    B stools characteristically do not contain red cells or leucocytes
    C pre-existing antibodies to rotavirus in the serum protects against the infection
    D it alters the cyclic AMP mechanism
    E breast milk provides a protection against rotavirus infection

21.8 **In Zellweger's syndrome:**
    A autosomal dominant inheritance occurs
    B the external ear is abnormal
    C abnormal calcification is a recognized feature
    D a significant increase in very long chain fatty acids in aminocytes is used to establish antenatal diagnosis
    E eye signs frequently occur in this disorder

21.9 **The following statements about porphyrias are correct:**
    A they are genetic disorders in which there are partial defects in the enzymes involved in haem synthesis
    B Δ-aminolaevulinic acid dehydrogenase deficiency is an autosomal dominant disorder
    C photosensitivity, haemolytic anaemia and splenomegaly are late childhood presentations
    D protoporphyrins are excreted in hepatic porphyrias
    E the disorder may mimic intra-abdominal surgical emergencies

21.7 A **True**   Rotaviral gastroenteritis is a common clinical
      B **True**   problem in the autumn and spring months. It affects
      C **False**   children aged between 6 months and 2 years. The
      D **False**   illness usually begins with fever, upper respiratory
      E **True**   symptoms and vomiting, followed by profuse watery
                       diarrhoea. As a result of dehydration and electrolyte
                       imbalance, the patients may develop neurological
                       symptoms. Rotavirus has been detected in the
                       stools of neonates and necrotizing entercolitis.
                       Extra-intestinal rotaviral infection affecting the liver
                       and kidney has been reported in immunocom-
                       promised children. The presence of rotaviral
                       particles in the stools can be confirmed by electron
                       microscopy.

21.8 A **False**   Zellweger's syndrome (cerebo-hepato-renal
      B **True**   syndrome) is an autosomal dominant disorder
      C **True**   characterized by the absence of peroxisomes and
      D **True**   defective function of peroxisomal enzymes. Patients
      E **True**   manifest with profound hypotonia dysmorphic
                       features, psychomotor retardation, sometimes
                       complicated by blindness and deafness. X-ray of the
                       knee shows calcific strippling of the patella. Prenatal
                       diagnosis using biochemical analysis of the
                       aminocytes has been developed.

21.9 A **True**   Porphyrias are disorders in haem synthesis. These
      B **False**   are generalized disorders but are classified as
      C **True**   hepatic or erythropoietic porphyrias. Partial defects
      D **False**   in the enzymes involved in haem synthesis lead to
      E **True**   clinical manifestations. Symptoms may be
                       precipitated by drugs, toxins and neoplasms. In all
                       except acute intermittent porphyria, photosensitivity
                       may occur. Presentation may be at any age.
                       Diagnosis is made on the basis of the urinary and
                       stool analysis of protoporphyrins. Specific enzyme
                       defects are identified in erythrocytes, skin fibroblasts
                       or liver biopsy specimens.

21.10 Correct statements regarding cholestatic jaundice in infancy include:
A extrahepatic atresia occurs in congenital heart disease
B α-1-antitrypsin deficiency is associated with intrahepatic cholestasis
C prognosis of arteriohepatic dysplasia is good
D the inheritance of lymphoedema with intrahepatic cholestasis is autosomal dominant
E septicaemia may cause intrahepatic cholestasis in infancy

21.11 The following statements about nutrition in liver disease are true:
A severe muscle wasting is seen
B reduction in midarm circumference occurs early in chronic liver disease
C absorption of medium chain triglycerides is minimally affected when the intraluminal bile concentration is low
D pancreatic function is affected in advanced liver disease
E the recommended energy allowance in advanced liver disease is 140–200% above the allowance for age

21.12 The following statements regarding pancreatitis are correct:
A it occurs in viral infections such as mumps
B haemorrhage and bruising are seen in severe attacks
C it is not seen in mucocutaneous lymph node syndrome
D pseudocyst formation is a recognized complication
E serum lipase activity remains high for less than 7 days

21.10 A **True** Cholestatic jaundice in infancy is a difficult clinical
B **True** problem. Many causes have been suggested but the
C **True** aetiology is often unknown. The prognosis is difficult
D **False** unless the cause is clearly known. Extrahepatic
E **True** atresia may lead to cholestasis but the exact
mechanism is not clear except in situations
associated with congenital abnormalities.
Intrahepatic cholestasis is often associated with a
known disorder, such as α-1-antitrypsin deficiency.
The prognosis is better in less severe forms of
cholestasis.

21.11 A **True** In chronic liver disease malnutrition occurs due to
B **True** maldigestion of fat, poor absorption of fat soluble
C **True** vitamins, and steatorrhoea due to the decrease of
D **False** intraduodenal bile salts. Later in the disease
E **True** gluconeogenesis is affected, leading to
hypoglycaemia and increased utilization of fat for
energy. The weight and growth pattern are
decreased and finally give rise to a picture of protein
energy malnutrition. The morbidity associated with
protein energy malnutrition includes developmental
delay, immune impairment and infection. Nutritional
support is important in chronic liver disease to
improve the outcome following liver transplantation.

21.12 A **True** Pancreatitis is seen in children following infections,
B **True** abdominal trauma, ingestion of drugs and also in
C **False** systemic disease. The children present with
D **True** abdominal pain, vomiting, fever and general ill
E **False** health. The pain increases in severity after 24–48
hours. In severe cases jaundice, ascites and pleural
effusion may occur. During this phase the pancreas
may become a necrotic, infected, inflammatory
mass. Investigations include full blood count, blood
sugar, calcium, serum amylase and serum lipase
along with electrolytes, and radiological
assessments are necessary in the management of
this disorder.

21.13 The following statements apply in protracted diarrhoea in infancy:
A It often follows acute infective diarrhoea
B stools may contain reducing substances
C it may be one of the features of child abuse
D congenital chloridorrhoea is a recognized cause
E osmotic and secretory diarrhoea are differentiated by stool analysis

21.14 Features that suggest a diagnosis of Crohn's disease are:
A bloody diarrhoea
B delayed skeletal maturation
C oxaluria
D normal faecal α-1-antitrypsin level
E abnormal liver function tests

21.15 In failure to thrive:
A the growth rate does not meet the growth potential that is expected for a child of that age
B muscle wasting is not a clinical sign
C psychosocial evaluation is essential in the management of this condition
D hospitalization may be necessary to determine whether the cause is organic or non-organic
E there may be an unrecognized problem of subdural haematoma following head injury

21.13 A **True**   Protracted diarrhoea in infancy is often a diagnostic
       B **True**   problem. Careful assessment of the infant is
       C **True**   essential to arrive at the diagnosis. There are
       D **True**   several causes, food sensitivity and post-enteritis
       E **True**   being the commonest. The infant loses weight due
                        to malabsorption. Coeliac disease, cystic fibrosis,
                        and some inborn errors of metabolism may present
                        as protracted diarrhoea. Up to 30% of cases may
                        not have an identifiable cause. Stool microbiological
                        assay is essential to exclude bacterial, viral and
                        parasitic pathogen. Management includes the
                        treatment of the cause where appropriate, dietary
                        manipulations to achieve adequate weight gain, as
                        well as relief of symptoms.

21.14 A **True**   Laboratory assessment involves the identification of
       B **True**   an infective cause of bloody diarrhoea. The full
       C **False**   blood count shows a picture suggestive of iron
       D **True**   deficiency anaemia and abnormal acute phase
       E **True**   reactants. There is thrombocytosis and low albumin.
                        Barium meal and follow-through helps in the
                        identification of areas of ulceration of the ileum. In
                        addition to the areas of thickening and fissuring of
                        the bowel wall, fistulae are seen in this examination
                        in Crohn's disease. Endoscopy with biopsy is the
                        most sensitive and specific test for evaluating
                        Crohn's ileocolitis.

21.15 A **True**   The management of failure to thrive is complex.
       B **False**   Failure to thrive usually describes a child often under
       C **True**   2 years of age with a weight gain pattern falling off
       D **True**   the percentile. Careful history, clinical examination,
       E **False**   observation of the child and the family will establish
                        a management plan appropriate for that particular
                        clinical situation. The organic causes may be due to
                        inadequate intake (cleft lip and palate, congenital
                        syndromes such as fetal alcohol syndrome). The
                        investigations would depend on the potential causes
                        from the history.

21.16 In cow's milk protein intolerance:
A the most common symptoms are vomiting, diarrhoea and poor weight gain
B jejunal biopsy reveals patchy partial villous atrophy
C older children may suffer from asthma
D explosive bloody diarrhoea and hypovolaemic shock are recognized complications
E stools may show reducing substances

21.17 The following laboratory investigations are indicated when coeliac disease is suspected:
A peripheral blood film
B serum triglycerides
C anti-gliadin, anti-reticulin and anti-endomysial antibodies
D urinary albumin
E stools for reducing substances

21.18 The following features suggest a diagnosis of coeliac disease:
A frequent, frothy, liquid foul-smelling stools
B intestinal obstruction in the neonatal period
C insidious onset of iron deficiency anaemia
D abdominal distension
E appearance of symptoms after the introduction of gluten containing foods on weaning

21.19 Features of pyloric stenosis include:
A profuse diarrhoea
B poor weight gain pattern
C poor feeding
D falling urinary output after the onset of the symptoms
E low serum bicarbonate

21.16　A　**True**　　Cow's milk protein intolerance commonly occurs in
　　　　B　**True**　　the first six months of life. Gastrointestinal symptoms
　　　　C　**True**　　are the commonest manifestation. Skin and
　　　　D　**True**　　respiratory manifestations have been observed.
　　　　E　**True**　　There is often a strong family history of atopic
　　　　　　　　　　　disorders. Withdrawing cow's milk from the diet may
　　　　　　　　　　　allow symptoms to subside within a few days. The
　　　　　　　　　　　symptoms will recur if the child is challenged with
　　　　　　　　　　　cow's milk after the child has been on a cow's milk
　　　　　　　　　　　free diet. IgE and radioallergosorbent tests are
　　　　　　　　　　　helpful in confirming the diagnosis.

21.17　A　**True**　　Laboratory analysis is non-specific in coeliac
　　　　B　**False**　 disease. However, anaemia, low albumin,
　　　　C　**True**　　cholesterol and vitamin A are all features suggestive
　　　　D　**False**　 of malabsorption. Stool fat analysis and xylose
　　　　E　**True**　　absorption tests are of value in assessing
　　　　　　　　　　　malabsorption. The serum antibodies to gliadin are
　　　　　　　　　　　used as screening tests for coeliac disease. Jejunal
　　　　　　　　　　　biopsy before and after the challenge with gliadin
　　　　　　　　　　　remains the confirmatory test for the diagnosis of
　　　　　　　　　　　coeliac disease.

12.18　A　**True**　　Coeliac disease causes malabsorption due to a
　　　　B　**False**　 defect in mucosal function which prevents the
　　　　C　**True**　　absorption of nutrients. The enteropathy is due to
　　　　D　**True**　　the sensitivity of the mucous membrane to the
　　　　E　**True**　　dietary protein gluten. The symptoms start when
　　　　　　　　　　　gluten containing food are introduced. Villous
　　　　　　　　　　　atrophy and crypt hyperplasia are seen on jejunal
　　　　　　　　　　　biopsy. Other malabsorption conditions, such as
　　　　　　　　　　　cow's milk protein intolerance, may give a similar
　　　　　　　　　　　microscopic appearance.

21.19　A　**False**　 Infants present with vomiting and hunger. A test feed
　　　　B　**True**　　may help to establish the diagnosis. Visible
　　　　C　**False**　 peristalsis may be seen during the test feed. The
　　　　D　**True**　　pyloric mass may or may not be palpable.
　　　　E　**False**　 Ultrasound of the tumour may help to establish the
　　　　　　　　　　　diagnosis. Metabolic disturbances may show a
　　　　　　　　　　　hypochloraemic alkalosis. Metabolic correction is
　　　　　　　　　　　necessary before surgical correction of the
　　　　　　　　　　　obstruction by pyloromyotomy. The prognosis is
　　　　　　　　　　　good.

21.20 The following statements regarding ulcerative colitis are correct:
  A growth retardation is uncommon
  B lower abdominal tenderness is a positive sign in the acute phase of the illness
  C tenesmus with lower abdominal pain is relieved by defaecation
  D there is increased risk of large intestinal adenocarcinoma in those with long standing disease
  E toxic megacolon is a recognized medical complication

21.21 Features suggestive of Hirschsprung's disease include:
  A abdominal distension
  B delay in passing meconium in the neonatal period
  C constipation followed by diarrhoea
  D normal rectal biopsy
  E hepatomegaly

21.22 The following features are encountered in food allergic colitis:
  A failure to thrive
  B frequent loose stools
  C normal mucosal pattern on colonoscopy
  D absence in exclusively breast fed babies
  E strong family history of atopy

21.20 A **True**   Ulcerative colitis is a chronic relapsing inflammatory
       B **True**   disease of the colon and the rectum. The inflamma-
       C **False**   tion is continuous and it is usually limited to the
       D **True**   colonic mucosa. The mucosal and submucosal
       E **True**   layers are infiltrated with inflammatory cells. The
                         cause of ulcerative colitis is unknown although an
                         immunological process is possible due to immune
                         complex activation and the evidence of antibodies.
                         The suppression of the symptoms with steroids and
                         immunosuppressives suggests the possibility of an
                         immune mechanism in the aetiology of the disease.

21.21 A **True**   Symptoms of Hirschsprung's disease often manifest
       B **True**   in the first few days of life. The short segment
       C **True**   disease may occur where the aganglionosis affects
       D **False**   the rectum with or without the sigmoid colon. It is
       E **False**   more common in males than in females. The long
                         segment disease affects males and females equally.
                         Histologically, there is absence of ganglions in the
                         myenteric plexus. Hirschsprung's enterocolitis has a
                         high mortality rate. Anomalies such as megaureter,
                         renal cyst disease and colonic polyposis are
                         associated with Hirchsprung's disease.

21.22 A **True**   Food allergic colitis is not an uncommon problem in
       B **True**   infancy. Several foods have been incriminated in this
       C **False**   disorder, and those commonly encountered include
       D **False**   cow's milk protein, eggs and soya proteins. Often
       E **True**   there is a strong family history. The definitive test is
                         elimination of the offending nutrient with rapid
                         resolution of the symptoms as well as signs. The
                         colonic mucosa also returns to normal appearance.
                         The condition is often underdiagnosed and mistaken
                         for other forms of colitis. Careful clinical assessment
                         and dietary evaluation is necessary to diagnose this
                         condition. A formal dietary challenge may be
                         necessary to confirm the diagnosis.

21.23 Ascites is a demonstrable clinical sign in the following conditions:
A hypothyroidism
B cirrhosis of the liver
C meconium peritonitis
D congenital cytomegaloviral infections
E mesenteric cysts

21.24 The following statements regarding intussusception in children are correct:
A it is a recognized problem in the first month of life
B the infant often passes partially formed stools early on in the illness
C the infant may appear well at the time of medical consultation
D the abdomen may appear scaphoid
E it is not seen in patients with cystic fibrosis

21.25 The following statements are true of constipation in children:
A it is a recognized cause of recurrent abdominal pain
B abdominal X-ray is of no value in the diagnosis of this condition
C it does not occur in children with cerebral palsy
D it may be diagnosed when urinary tract infections are investigated
E in the older child medical therapy alone achieves satisfactory results

21.23 A **True**   Ascites is the accumulation of fluid in the peritoneal
       B **True**   cavity. The pathogenesis of ascites is explained by
       C **True**   two theories. In the underfill theory, the hydrostatic
       D **True**   pressure increases in the hepatosplanchnic
       E **False**   circulation. Hypoalbuminaemia due to the liver
                      disease and sodium retention in the intravascular
                      compartment contribute to the leakage of fluid into
                      the peritoneal cavity. In the overflow theory sodium
                      is retained to maintain the oncotic pressure,
                      increasing the hydrostatic pressure in the
                      hepatosplanchnic circulation with leakage of fluid
                      into the peritoneal cavity.

21.24 A **False**   Intussusception is a common cause of intestinal
       B **True**   obstruction in children aged between 3 months and
       C **True**   1 year. The condition is more common in boys than
       D **True**   in girls. Most infants are healthy and well nourished.
       E **False**   Many have signs and symptoms of an upper
                      respiratory tract infection. The infants have a painful
                      cry, drawing up of the knees and appear pale.
                      Vomiting is a common sign. A recognizable feature
                      at surgery is inflamed lymphoid glands, enlarged
                      Peyer's patches, presumably due to a viral infection.
                      In the older children, anatomical abnormalities such
                      as Meckel's diverticulum, polyps on the intestinal
                      wall and enteric cyst have been noted.

21.25 A **True**   Constipation is a cause for a paediatric consultation.
       B **False**   There are several organic causes for constipation
       C **False**   and these are identified in the history and clinical
       D **True**   examination. The symptom does not only affect the
       E **False**   child, but also the parents psychologically. Most
                      children with chronic constipation present in the
                      preschool years. In these children it is unlikely an
                      organic cause is present. Abdominal pain and
                      occasional nausea and vomiting may be the
                      symptoms which attract medical attention. If an
                      organic cause is not obvious during the consultation,
                      psychological support is indicated.

22. Diabetes

22.1 The following statements apply in the diet of children with diabetes mellitus:
  A the nutritional intake should be adjusted to the insulin intake
  B a very strict dietary regime should be followed
  C regular assessment of the diet is appropriate
  D the energy requirement is calculated on the number of calories/body weight
  E strict adherence to a diet in schoolchildren could lead to rebellious tendencies and major psychological problems

22.2 To achieve optimal control, the following statements apply in the long-term management of diabetes with insulin:
  A the insulin dosage remains the same throughout the toddler age group
  B twice-daily insulin gives satisfactory results
  C pen devices are acceptable in some instances
  D the diet must be matched to the insulin dose and frequency
  E a mixture of long acting and intermediate acting insulins has made management easier in some children

22.3 The following are the usual recommendations for the diet of children with insulin dependent diabetes mellitus (IDDM):
  A the average intake should be 125% in excess of the normal intake
  B the carbohydrate intake should be 40–50% of the total energy intake
  C the protein intake should be restricted
  D micronutrients should be added as supplements
  E vitamin supplements are not necessary
  F the intake should be considered in the form of portions and should be distributed at fixed times during the day

22.1 A **False**   In the management of children with diabetes mellitus
     B **False**   the nutritional requirement is very similar to other
     C **True**   children. Diabetic children are advised to follow
     D **False**   guidelines, but no strict regime should be instituted.
     E **True**   The nutrient intake must be adjusted to the needs of
                     the child and his/her activities and age rather than to
                     the blood sugar pattern. The dietary intake increases
                     as soon as treatment with insulin has started. It also
                     fluctuates with the different age groups. The
                     dietician plays a key role in doing dietary assess-
                     ments at regular intervals. The establishment of a
                     multidisciplinary team in the care of the child is
                     essential in order to look into the psychosocial
                     needs and the monitoring of injections.

22.2 A **False**   Several insulin preparations are available in the
     B **True**   management of insulin dependent diabetes mellitus
     C **True**   (IDDM). The standard beef and pork mixes are still
     D **False**   available but have the disadvantage of being
     E **True**   antigenic. The purified pork insulin and the human
                     insulin are produced by recombinant DNA
                     technology using *Escherichia coli* or semi-
                     synthetically. The human insulin may have a shorter
                     duration of action than the pork insulin in some
                     children. Recent reports suggest an increased
                     incidence of asymptomatic hypoglycaemia so
                     patients should be closely monitored especially
                     when they are on twice-daily doses of a mixture of
                     short acting and intermediary acting insulins. The
                     three main types of insulin preparation are:
                     – short acting: relatively rapid onset of action,
                       soluble
                     – intermediary acting
                     – long acting: slower onset of action, longer duration

22.3 A **False**   The dietary requirement in children with diabetes
     B **True**   mellitus should be adjusted to their activities, age,
     C **False**   family lifestyle and growth pattern. It is
     D **False**   recommended that the energy requirement should
     E **True**   be the same as for diabetic patients and 40–50%
     F **False**   should come in the form of carbohydrate with
                     30–35% in the form of fat. It is not necessary to have
                     added sodium, added vitamins or micronutrients in
                     the diet. It is essential that the distribution of energy
                     is among carbohydrates, fats and proteins, and the
                     meals are adjusted according to the child's activities,
                     age, lifestyle and growth pattern.

22.4 The following statements regarding hypoglycaemia are correct:
A glucose is the most important source of energy for the brain
B it alters the cerebral blood flow
C it decreases the rate of acetylcholine turnover resulting in cerebral dysfunction
D the receptors for amino acids, such as N-methyl-D-aspartate receptors, are often affected
E fructose 1–6 diphosphatase deficiency is a recognized cause

22.5 The following must be considered in the management of diabetic ketoacidosis:
A dietary assessment in the previous 24 hours
B duration of the symptoms
C blood gas results before commencing i.v. fluid regimes
D precise monitoring and record keeping
E regular monitoring of urea, electrolytes, blood sugars and plasma bicarbonate every 2–4 hours in the early stages
F correction of the blood glucose to normal levels

22.6 Recognized complications in diabetes mellitus include:
A recurrent infection
B growth failure
C retinopathy within 2 years of developing diabetes
D reduced pupillary adaptation to darkness
E asymptomatic hypoglycaemia
F poor school performance

22.4 A True   There is no clear definition of hypoglycaemia. It is
      B True   not a diagnosis in itself and it has many causes.
      C True   There is no doubt that prolonged recurrent
      D True   symptomatic hypoglycaemic episodes can result in
      E True   permanent brain damage. Glucose is an important
                 energy source in brain metabolism and several
                 animal model studies have shown that it alters the
                 cerebral circulation. It could also alter the enzyme
                 activities in the brain thereby affecting the release of
                 chemical transmitters as well as activities of the
                 membranes.

22.5 A False   In the management of ketoacidosis, standard
      B False   protocols adapted for local needs are essential. The
      C False   principles of the standard protocols should include:
      D True   – assessment of the severity (acidosis, level of
      E True   hydration)
      F False   – precise monitoring and record keeping (flow chart
                   of results, ECG)
                 – good i.v. access
                 – urgent restoration of circulating volume
                 – gradual reversal of hypoglycaemia plus replace-
                   ment of fluids and deficit together with the daily
                   fluid requirement
                 – close monitoring of blood glucose, serum sodium,
                   potassium and bicarbonate
                 – neurological observations, e.g. the state of
                   consciousness, pulse, BP, signs of raised
                   intracranial pressure

22.6 A False   The development of overt complications in IDDM in
      B True   children is poorly understood. However,
      C False   hypoglycaemic episodes, poor growth patterns, poor
      D True   school and educational performance are well-
      E True   recognized problems. Other endocrine glands can
      F True   be affected due to an autoimmune process. The
                 development of microalbuminaemia may be an early
                 sign of nephropathy. The value of detecting
                 microalbuminuria and the development of other
                 clinical signs such as hypertension and its
                 management is not clearly understood. However,
                 monitoring growth pattern in childhood is essential
                 as is regular direct ophthalmoscopy at least once a
                 year in adolescence.

22.7 **In insulin dependent diabetes mellitus (IDDM):**
A most children with recent onset IDDM have had symptoms over 6 months
B weight loss is not a classical feature
C urinary retention is an early feature
D diabetic ketoacidosis is a well-recognized presentation
E metabolic disturbance is more common in younger age groups

22.8 **The following statements about the pathogenesis of diabetes are correct:**
A most recent studies have shown that there is an increasing incidence of diabetes in many countries
B The histocompatibility markers (HLA) DR3 and DR4 are associated with an increased risk of developing type I diabetes mellitus
C transient neonatal diabetes mellitus classically occurs in small-for-date infants
D radiation is one of the most important environmental factors in the causation of diabetes
E there is a strong association between the onset of diabetes and Coxsackie B10 infection

22.9 **The following statements regarding the eyes and children with IDDM are correct:**
A pupillary dilatation to darkness is a form of assessment of diabetic control
B pupillary diameter is smaller than in children of the same age group who have no diabetes
C diabetic retinopathy is rare
D the ophthalmic damage of the iris is not reversible despite improved control
E intensive therapy in diabetic control helps to improve the neuropathy

22.10 **Chronic effects of IDDM include:**
A joint dysfunction
B recurring hypoglycaemia
C metabolic control preventing the onset of nephropathy
D early onset hypertension accelerating the progress of nephropathy
E smoking aggravating the macrovascular complications in diabetes

22.7 A **False** Most children with IDDM present with polyuria,
B **False** polydypsia, polyphagia and weight loss and often
C **False** complain of lethargy. The parents may notice that
D **True** the children's behaviour and activity diminishes
E **True** rapidly. When metabolic decompensation occurs they present in a life-threatening situation with severe diabetic ketoacidosis. Most children with recent onset IDDM have had symptoms for less than 1 month and present with the classical features listed above.

22.8 A **True** The pathogenesis of the onset type I diabetes
B **True** mellitus is a complex one. Various studies have
C **True** clearly shown that genetic factors as well as
D **False** environmental factors lead to diabetes. Transient
E **True** neonatal diabetes mellitus may be associated with the development of late onset IDDM.

22.9 A **True**
B **True**
C **True**
D **False**
E **True**

22.10 A **True** The autoimmune disease process affecting the
B **False** thyroid gland has been reported in IDDM after the
C **True** child has had diabetes for over 5 years. Joint
D **True** dysfunction is a well-recognized complication, which
E **True** occurs as a result of the glycosylation of the proteins of the tissues around the joints. Often joint dysfunction may be associated with other problems such as retinopathy and nephropathy. Nephropathy may lead to hypertension and eventually to end stage renal disease and the patient may require renal dialysis or transplantation. 30–40% of patients with IDDM are likely to develop end stage renal disease after approximately 15–20 years of the disease. Good metabolic control is extremely important in order to prevent nephropathy.

23. Genetics

23.1 Which of the following statements apply in the expression of a gene:
   A both the alleles must be identical for the expression of a feature
   B in uniparental disomy there are three genes but during early cell division one is lost, resulting in meiosis
   C in Angelman's syndrome, the division occurs on chromosome 15 of maternal origin
   D in the Prader-Willi syndrome the deletion of chromosome 15 occurs in both
   E lyonization may allow the expression of an X-linked disease in females

23.2 The following statements apply to the DNA structure:
   A the sugar in DNA is sucrose
   B the phosphate bonds link the sugar molecule
   C the four bases in the structure are adenine, cytosine, guanine and thymine
   D change in the pH could produce a single stranded DNA
   E the majority of the DNA is in the mitochondria

23.3 Recognized features of Down syndrome include:
   A AV canal malformation
   B distal palmar triradii
   C atlanto-axial instability
   D cleft lip and palate
   E rocker-bottom feet

23.1   A   **False**
       B   **True**
       C   **False**
       D   **False**
       E   **True**

23.2   A   **False**   The DNA consists of the deoxyribose sugar
       B   **True**   molecules which are repeatedly combined with the
       C   **True**   phosphate molecules to provide the strands of DNA.
       D   **True**   There are four bases which link the deoxyribose
       E   **False**   sugar. The two strands of DNA are held together by
                        the hydrogen bonds between the bases, namely
                        adenine and thymine, and cytosine and guanine.
                        The double helix may be disrupted by heat and
                        changes in the pH. Change in the heat or the pH
                        could restore the double-stranded DNA molecule.
                        Most of the DNA is in the nucleus but a very small
                        amount is in the mitochondria.

23.3   A   **True**   Recognized features of Down syndrome are short
       B   **True**   stature, typical craniofacial composition such as
       C   **True**   microencephaly, brachycephaly, upslanting of the
       D   **False**   palpebral fissures, inner epicanthic folds, speckling
       E   **False**   of the iris (Brushfield's spots), small nose, low nasal
                        bridge, small ears with small or absent ear lobes, flat
                        facial profile, short neck, mouth held open with
                        tongue protruding, hypotonia, brachydactyly, short
                        hands and fingers, single flexion crease on the 5th
                        finger (incurving of the little finger of the hands).
                        Congenital heart disease occurs in between one-
                        third and one-half of the cases with endocardial
                        cushion defects, VSD being the most common.

23.4 Recognized features of Patau syndrome include:
A Brushfield's spots
B clinodactyly
C cleft palate
D polydactyly
E scalp defects

23.5 The following are correct statements regarding genes in paediatric malignancies:
A an identifiable gene is recognized in all paediatric malignancies
B in Down syndrome there is a higher occurrence of leukaemia, testicular tumours and retinoblastoma
C osteosarcoma is seen in XYY disorders
D the gene locus for retinoblastoma is on chromosome 13
E retinoblastoma occurs in hereditary and non-hereditary forms

23.6 Genetic features of thalassaemias include:
A homozygous thalassaemia causes mild disease
B the affected gene is the β-globin gene
C a number of different mutations are seen in different ethnic groups
D antenatal diagnosis is made by chorionic villus sampling
E the mutations are all polynucleotide substitutions

23.7 Features of the genetics of the fragile X chromosome include:
A affected males are normally retarded
B the X chromosomes contain a break at the distal end of the long arm
C the affected individual may develop autism
D female carriers are clinically unaffected
E expansion of the trinucleotide (CGG) on the X chromosome gives rise to the permutation and the individual is clinically normal

23.4 A False   The cardinal features of Patau syndrome (trisomy
      B False   13) include intrauterine growth retardation,
      C True   microcephaly, structural malformations of the brain,
      D True   altered facial appearance, hypotelorism, a small
      E True   nose, a cleft lip and palate. In the limbs, post-axial
                   polydactyly of the hands and feet, flexion
                   contractures and rocker-bottom feet may also be
                   present. The other associated abnormalities could
                   be renal as well as cardiac which are frequent. The
                   sequence of malformations affecting the brain are
                   known as holoprosencephaly. Normally, the
                   forebrain divides into two hemispheres and the optic
                   vesicles develop to form the eyes. In
                   holoprosencephaly the forebrain divides
                   incompletely and the optic vesicles develop in close
                   proximity leading to hypotelorism or cyclopia.

23.5 A False   Cancers usually occur as a result of somatic gene
      B True   mutation or failure of gene regulation. Genetic
      C True   instability and DNA repair disorders may be
      D True   associated with certain malignancies such as
      E True   squamous cell carcinoma in xeroderma pigmentosa
                   (autosomal recessive disorder). There are
                   recognized malignancies in chromosomal disorders.
                   Molecular genetic analysis has been useful in
                   detecting haematological malignancies.

23.6 A False   All β-thalassaemia defects involve the DNA
      B True   sequence of the β-globin gene. This leads to an
      C True   abnormal expression of the gene. Mutations may
      D True   occur on the exon or the intron portion of the gene.
      E False   This affects the processing of the RNA to form
                   mRNA. When this is transported into the cytoplasm
                   it affects the synthesis of the globin.

23.7 A True   Fragile X syndrome is a condition where a
      B True   nonclassical mutation produces a genetic disease.
      C True   Some of these mutations lead to an unusual non-
      D True   Mendelian inheritance. These mutations are
      E True   unstable. Expansion of nucleotide repeat sequences
                   is responsible for this condition. In the region of the
                   chromosome X where there is a break, there is a
                   lack of expression of a gene (familial mental
                   retardation – 1 or FMR-1) and inappropriate
                   methylation, with a marked expansion of the
                   trinucleotide repeat (CGG).

23.8 Principles in the techniques of hybridization include:
A insertion of a DNA sequence into a plasmid is used in dot blot analysis
B enzymatic amplification of a particular DNA sequence is used in polymerase chain reaction
C the polymerase chain reactions are used for detection of single nucleotide changes in the DNA and analysis of restriction fragment length polymorphisms
D dot blot analysis is used for polymerase chain products
E southern blot analysis is used for the detection of a trisomy

23.9 The following are the appropriate tissue sources for DNA analysis for diagnosis in single gene disorders:
A whole blood is required for carrier detection and postnatal genetic studies
B buccal mucosa washings are useful for antenatal diagnosis
C chorionic villus sampling is preferable to amniocentesis for the diagnosis of single gene disorders
D maternal skin biopsy is necessary for the diagnosis of Duchenne muscular dystrophy
E blood and tissue sample for retrospective diagnosis is helpful in single gene disorders

23.10 The following statements apply in the prenatal diagnosis of single gene disorders by DNA analysis:
A restriction fragment length analysis is utilized in the diagnosis of neurofibromatosis
B oligonucleotide analysis is useful for α-1-antitrypsin deficiency
C it is not applicable in the diagnosis of cystic fibrosis
D prenatal diagnosis of insulin dependent diabetes mellitus may be undertaken
E the degree of accuracy for diagnosis is high in couples identified as being at risk for retinoblastoma

23.8 A False
      B True
      C True
      D True
      E False

23.9 A True
      B False
      C True
      D False
      E True

23.10 A True   In single gene disorders it is essential that a clear
      B True   history, examination (where applicable) and family
      C False   history is taken before DNA analysis. Where there is
      D False   a marker case in the family it is helpful to take
      E True   samples of blood from the affected individual as well
                  as both parents. This will enable the family to be
                  counselled. This technique has been used in the
                  antenatal diagnosis of several conditions.

24. Cardiology

24.1 The following statements about rheumatic fever are correct:
- A the heart is the only organ affected
- B it usually follows an upper respiratory tract infection
- C it commonly affects the mitral or aortic valves
- D symptoms of mitral incompetence develop within 2–4 years
- E apical systolic cardiac murmur radiating to the axilla accompanied by a muffled first heart sound may be the first sign of cardiac involvement

24.2 The following statements concerning persistent common atrioventricular (AV) canal defects are correct:
- A different types of malformations occur
- B patients with complete AV canal defects are prone to frequent respiratory tract infections
- C Down syndrome is frequently associated with endocardial cushion defects
- D a systolic thrill is present when there is mitral regurgitation
- E the M-mode echocardiogram shows an enlarged right ventricle and paradoxical movement of the interventricular septum

24.3 An abnormal electrocardiogram rhythm strip may detect:
- A Wolff-Parkinson-White syndrome
- B a long QT interval
- C left ventricular hypertrophy
- D rheumatic heart disease
- E hypertrophic cardiomyopathy

24.1 A **False** Rheumatic fever affects other organs such as the
     B **True**   blood vessels, joints, central nervous system and
     C **True**   subcutaneous tissues. The illness follows an upper
     D **False** respiratory tract infection caused by β-haemolytic
     E **True**   streptococci group A. Rheumatic fever is thought to be an autoimmune disease. Non-specific lesions resulting from fibroid degeneration involve the connective tissue and the specific lesions. Aschoff's nodules affect the paravascular tissues. In the heart all three layers are affected (pancarditis) and the cardiac involvement may be in the acute or chronic stage.

24.2 A **True**   Persistent common atrioventricular canal defects
     B **True**   include atrial septal defects (ASDs) of the primum
     C **True**   type, ventricular septal defects and atrioventricular
     D **True**   valve defects. The clinical manifestations can vary
     E **True**   from those similar to a large ASD, as in patients with ostium primum ASD and minimal insufficiency of the AV valve, to those with complete AV canal defects where they develop symptoms of congestive heart failure in early infancy. Auscultatory manifestations may vary as the intensity of the heart sounds varies, along with a systolic murmur. The murmur may be easily audible at the apex radiating to the lower left sternal border. Cardiac enlargement may be present on the chest radiograph.

24.3 A **True**   Rhythm strips in ECGs are mainly used for the
     B **True**   diagnosis of the Wolff-Parkinson-White syndrome
     C **False** and a long QT interval. The findings of an ECG
     D **False** should be interpreted in the context of the clinical
     E **False** situation. In the Wolff-Parkinson-White syndrome, the PR interval is short for the age of the patient, there is slurred upstroke to the QRS complex as well as changes to the ST or T waves. A prolonged QT interval is diagnosed when the correct QT interval is longer than 0.44 (i.e. QT interval in seconds/square root of the PR interval in seconds).

24.4 **The following statements about atrial septal defects (ASDs) are true:**
   A small ASDs are due to incompetence of the valve of the foramen ovale
   B multiple defects may occur in the region of the floor of fossa ovalis
   C large ASDs often lead to atrial dysrhythmias in later life
   D incomplete right bundle branch block is a result of a conduction defect
   E fixed splitting of the second sound is a characteristic auscultatory feature

24.5 **Features commonly encountered in children with middle aortic syndrome include:**
   A diminished femoral pulses
   B cyanosis at birth
   C clinical manifestation at 14 years of age
   D hypertension
   E medical treatment is satisfactory in most cases

24.6 **The following are cyanotic congenital cardiac lesions:**
   A patent ductus arteriosus
   B cor triatriatum
   C L-corrected transposition
   D anomalous innominate arteries
   E pulmonary atresia with a ventricular septal defect

24.7 **The following statements about myocarditis in childhood are correct:**
   A it may go unrecognized in children with viral illness
   B it is seen often in children with congenital heart disease
   C Coxsackie B virus infection is often the virus responsible in epidemics
   D there is a decrease in cardiac end diastolic volume
   E fibroblasts are seen in the myocardium in the healing stages

24.4 A **True**   Congenital ASDs are common. They may be
      B **True**   isolated or in combination with other defects. When
      C **True**   there are associated defects the clinical presentation
      D **False**   is often in early infancy or neonatal period. The true
      E **True**   defects are those in the region of the fossa ovalis.
                      The size of the defects vary. The clinical signs
                      depend on the age of the child and the presence of
                      an associated anomaly. Moderate to large shunts
                      are associated with a pulmonary systolic murmur.

24.5 A **False**   Middle aortic syndrome is a recognized condition
      B **False**   presenting between the ages of 2 months and 14
      C **True**   years. The common clinical presentations include
      D **True**   asymptomatic hypertension, severe headaches,
      E **True**   nose bleeds and cardiac failure. This is an
                      uncommon condition that can cause severe
                      hypertension with a risk of life-threatening
                      complications. It has been described in children with
                      William's syndrome. It may be mistaken for
                      coarctation of the aorta but in coarctation the
                      femoral pulses are not easily palpable.

24.6 A **False**
      B **True**
      C **False**
      D **False**
      E **True**

24.7 A **True**   Myocarditis (inflammation of the muscular wall of the
      B **False**   heart muscle) is rare in children. The disease may
      C **True**   go undiagnosed in some children, whilst in others it
      D **False**   may cause sudden death. The commonest cause in
      E **True**   children is viral but other agencies such as bacterial,
                      protozoal, fungal (*Candida*), drugs (tetracycline,
                      isoniazide) and autoimmune reactions have been
                      identified. An immunological basis for the
                      progression of the disease has been identified both
                      on autopsy findings and animal models. Microscopic
                      changes are non-specific and macroscopically the
                      heart weight is increased. The muscle is pale and
                      flabby and petechial haemorrhages are seen on the
                      epicardial surface of the myocardium. Pericardial
                      effusion is not an uncommon finding. Myocardial
                      function is usually reduced in the presence of
                      extensive interstitial inflammation or injury.

24.8 Clinical presentations of myocarditis in children include:
  A rapid weight loss along with symptoms of upper respiratory tract infection
  B serious ill health in neonates
  C a pansystolic murmur at the apex
  D muffled heart sounds in the presence of pericarditis
  E a previously well child who presents with cardiac failure

24.9 The following statements regarding cardiomyopathy are correct:
  A it must be considered in patients who present with supraventricular tachycardia
  B valvular disease is often a feature
  C idiopathic dilated cardiomyopathy is commoner in males than females
  D congestive cardiac failure is a rare presentation of endocardial fibroelastosis
  E medical treatment is effective in endomyocardial fibrosis

24.10 The following statements apply in children with infective endocarditis:
  A they have underlying heart disease
  B they have an audible heart murmur
  C in the neonate the clinical picture may be that of overwhelming sepsis
  D the erythrocyte sedimentation rate is always high
  E Osler's nodes are diagnostic features

24.11 The following are true of total anomalous pulmonary venous connections:
  A a major cardiac defect is often associated with the infracardiac type
  B cyanosis is a common finding and mixing of blood occurs in the right atrium
  C murmurs are infrequently audible in cases with obstruction
  D feeding difficulties are common in cases with a restrictive interatrial communication
  E surgery is indicated in patients who are symptomatic in the neonatal period

24.8 A True   The clinical presentation of myocarditis varies with
      B True   age and immune status. It is a recognized cause in
      C True   sudden infant death syndrome. Myocarditis may
      D True   occur in children with hepatitis or encephalitis. The
      E True   clinical features are more severe in neonates. Often
               the illness commences with mild upper respiratory
               tract symptoms and low grade temperature.

24.9 A True   Cardiomyopathy affects the ventricular myocardium
      B False   of the heart where there is a structural or functional
      C False   abnormality. These patients do not have raised
      D False   blood pressure, congenital heart disease, pulmonary
      E False   vascular disease or coronary heart disease. The
               cardiomyopathies may be primary or secondary. The
               primary cardiomyopathies may be dilated,
               hypertrophic or restrictive.

24.10 A True   Infective endocarditis is a recognized complication of
      B True   congenital heart disease. The endocardium, valves
      C True   or related structures may be infected by bacterial,
      D False   fungal, chlamydial or viral organisms. The children
      E False   may be acutely ill or may be identified after several
               months. Heart murmurs are classic findings. There
               may be accompanying non-specific symptoms
               affecting other systems. Laboratory investigations
               are essential and several blood cultures may be
               necessary to identify the causative organism.
               Echocardiography is increasingly used to confirm
               the diagnosis. Use of prophylactic antibiotics in high-
               risk cases is standard medical practice.

24.11 A True   Total anomalous pulmonary venous connection
      B True   occurs when pulmonary veins connect anomalously
      C True   to the systemic venous circulation. There are four
      D True   types, classified according to the site of connection:
      E True   supracardiac, cardiac, infracardiac and mixed.
               Symptoms depend on the types of connection,
               obstruction to the connection, size of the interatrial
               communication and other associated anomalies. The
               diagnostic investigations are echocardiogram and
               catheter studies.

24.12 In the treatment of infective endocarditis:
  A oral antibiotics given for 4–6 weeks produce a satisfactory response
  B regular blood cultures are indicated after therapy begins
  C vancomycin is the drug of choice when the organism is methicillin resistant *Staphylococcus aureus*
  D minimum duration of treatment with antibiotics is often more than 6 weeks
  E surgery is indicated when there is severe congestive heart failure

24.13 Features of mitral valve prolapse include:
  A chest pain
  B clinical manifestation in the neonatal period
  C cyanosis
  D arrhythmias in the first year of life
  E thrombotic episodes are rare

24.14 The following statements regarding patent ductus arteriosus are true:
  A isolated patent ductus arteriosus may produce symptoms in the preterm infant in the second week of extrauterine life
  B increased arterial concentration of oxygen causes constriction of the muscles of the wall of the ductus arteriosus
  C in critical pulmonary stenosis in the neonate the duct patency is essential to improve the pulmonary blood flow
  D the clinical sign of a murmur may be detected when a child is examined during a chest infection
  E the pulse volume is normal in affected children

24.15 The following statements about supraventricular tachycardia in children are correct:
  A the rate of often over 230 beats per minute
  B normal P waves occur before the QRS complexes
  C it may be confused with sinus tachycardia
  D it is a recognized arrhythmia in the Wolff-Parkinson-White syndrome
  E the diving reflex always reverts back to sinus rhythm

24.12 A **False**   Management of bacterial endocarditis includes the
       B **True**   appropriate use of antibiotics, isolation of the
       C **True**   organism, assessment of regurgitant murmurs or
       D **True**   embolic episodes, and control of fatigue. Surgery
       E **True**   has been an adjunct to medical treatment especially when there is congestive cardiac failure, persistent infection or embolization.

24.13 A **True**   A murmur and a midsystolic click are the typical
       B **False**   auscultatory findings in mitral valve prolapse. The
       C **False**   click and the murmur vary depending on the position
       D **False**   of the patient. The findings also vary after exercise.
       E **False**   A small subgroup of patients may be symptomatic and suffer chest pain, weakness, palpitations, dyspnoea, dizziness, syncope, anxiety and orthstatic hypotension. The electrocardiogram is usually normal as is the chest radiograph. An echocardiogram is useful.

24.14 A **True**   The patent ductus is a normal structure in the fetus
       B **True**   and closes soon after birth in the newborn. Closure
       C **True**   of the duct occurs as a result of the circulatory
       D **True**   changes and lung expansion immediately after birth.
       E **False**   The increase in concentration of the oxygen in the blood causes vasoconstriction of the duct. The high concentration of the prostaglandin degradation products enhances the closure. Congenital infections such as rubella in the first trimester frequently results in the persistence of the ductus. The child may be asymptomatic and the continuous murmur may be the only clinical sign. The treatment of the ductus may be supportive or definitive. Supportive therapy is necessary when the child is symptomatic. Umbrella closure via the transcatheter technique has been developed as a definitive procedure.

24.15 A **True**   Supraventricular tachycardia is an abnormally rapid
       B **True**   rhythm that originates proximal to the bifurcation of
       C **True**   the bundle of His. There are no flutter waves on the
       D **True**   ECG. The rate is often over 230 per minute and in
       E **False**   infants over 300 per minute. The QRS complexes during the attack are identical to the QRS complexes in sinus rhythm. It may be difficult to identify the P waves. Sympathomimetic drugs may precipitate an attack.

Index

Abdominal pain, recurrent, 149, 150
Absence seizures, 81, 82
Achondroplasia, 99, 100
Adenosine, 107, 108
   deaminase deficiency, 49, 50
Adenovirus infection, 13, 14
Adrenal hyperplasia, congenital, 3, 4, 5, 6
Adrenal hypoplasia, congenital, 1, 2
AIDS, lungs in, 111, 112
Allergy
   colitis and, 159, 160
   peanut, 47, 48
Anaemia, iron deficiency, 65, 66
Anomalous pulmonary venous connections, total, 179, 180
Anorexia nervosa, 89, 90
Anterior spinal artery syndrome, 83, 84
Antibiotics, 105, 106
   macrolide, 103, 104
Anticonvulsants, 103, 104
Antituberculous drugs, adverse effects of, 127, 128
Antiviral agents, 109, 110
Apgar scale, criteria used in, 27, 28
Apnoea in preterm infants, causes of, 23, 24
Apparent life-threatening events, 113, 114
Arthralgia, causes of, 97, 98
Arthritis
   pauciarticular juvenile chronic, 93, 94
   psoriatic, 97, 98
Arthrogryphosis multiplex congenita, 97, 98
Ascites, 161, 162
Asthma
   complications, 117, 118
   devices for different age groups, 107, 108
   inhaled steroids for, 119, 120
   mechanisms in, 113, 114
   pathological process in, 117, 118
   pathology of, 119, 120
   risk of developing, 119, 120
Ataxia
   acute, 77, 78
   Friedreich's, 85, 86
Atrial septal defects, 176, 177, 178
Atrioventricular canal defects, persistent
   common, 175, 176
Autoantibodies and disease, 99, 100

BCG vaccination, 39, 40
Biliary atresia, extrahepatic, 147, 148
Blood count, normal preterm, 35, 36
Bone disease, neonatal metabolic, 29, 30
Brain death, 81, 82
Bronchial hyperreactivity, 117, 118
Bronchiectasis, 115, 116
Bronchiolitis, 111, 112
   acute, 113, 114
Bronchoscopy in children, 123, 124
Bruises, ageing of, 57, 58
Burns, non-accidental injury and, 57, 58

Calcitonin, 10
Calcium/phosphorus metabolism, 9, 10
Cancers, genes in paediatric, 171, 172
Candidiasis, chronic mucocutaneous, 49, 50
Cardiogenesis, 131, 132
Cardiology, 175–82
Cardiomyopathy, 179, 180
Cell biology, 43, 44
Central value, measures of, 101, 102
Cerebral palsy diplegia, 85, 86

Cerebrospinal fluid, 83, 84
Child abuse, 55–8
Children's Act, 91–2
Cholestatic jaundice, 153, 154
Chronic fatigue syndrome, 89, 90
Cisapride, 103, 104
Coagulation deficiencies, 61, 62
Coeliac disease, 157, 158
Cold stress, 33, 34
Colitis, food allergic, 159, 160
Congenital infections, causes of, 11, 12
Congenital pulmonary lymphangiectasis, 121, 122
Constipation, 161, 162
Convulsions, febrile, 79, 80
Cord hemisection, 83, 84
Cow's milk protein intolerance, 157, 158
Craniopharyngioma, 63, 64
Crohn's disease, 149, 150, 155, 156
Croup, 121, 122
Cushing's disease, 7, 8
Cyanotic congenital cardiac lesions, 177, 178
Cystic fibrosis, 149, 150
    DNase therapy in, 109, 110
    gene, 115, 116
    hyponatraemia and, 71, 72
    problems in, 115, 116
Cytokines, 47, 48

Depression, 89, 90
Dermatology, 51–4
Dermatomyositis, 95, 96
Development, 37–8
Diabetes insipidus, nephrogenic, 9, 10
Diabetes mellitus, 163–8
    chronic effects of IDDM, 167, 168
    complications in, 165, 166
    diet and, 163, 164
    eyes and IDDM, 167, 168
    hypoglycaemia, 165, 166
    insulin and, 163, 164
    ketoacidosis, 165, 166, 167, 168
    pathogenesis of, 167, 168
    presenting features, 167, 168
Diarrhoea
    protracted, 155, 156
    rotavirus, 151, 152
Dispersion, measures of, 101, 102
Diuretics, 105, 106
DNA, 43, 44
    analysis, 173, 174
    structure, 169, 170

DNase therapy in cystic fibrosis, 109, 110
Down syndrome, 169, 170
Drowning, salt water, 77, 78
Drug abuse, adolescent, 89, 90
Duchenne muscular dystrophy, 85, 86

Ehlers-Danlos syndrome, 51, 52
Electrocardiogram rhythm strips, 175, 176
Embryology, 129–36
Endocarditis, infective, 179, 180
    treatment of, 181, 182
Endocrinology, 1–10
Enterocolitis, necrotizing see necrotizing enterocolitis
Eosinophilia, peripheral blood, 59, 60
Epstein-Barr virus, 17, 18
Erythema neonatorum, 53, 54
Eyes
    development of, 133, 134
    IDDM and, 167, 168

Familial Mediterranean fever, 17, 18
Fatigue syndrome, chronic, 89, 90
Febrile convulsions, 79, 80
Fertilization, 131, 132
Fetal development, 32
    immune mechanisms and date of, 47, 48
Fetomaternal circulation, 129, 130
Fistula, tracheo-oesophageal, 33, 34
'Floppy baby', causes of, 23, 24
Fractures, child abuse and, 55, 56
Fragile X chromosome, 171, 172
Friedreich's ataxia, 85, 86

Galactosaemia, 69, 70
Gametogenesis, 131, 132
Gastroenterology, 147–62
Gastrointestinal tract, development of, 133, 134
Gastro-oesophageal reflux, 147, 148
Gaucher's disease, 69, 70
Genetics, 169–74
    expressions of a gene, 169, 170
    genes in paediatric malignancies, 171, 172
    single gene disorders, 173, 174
Genital system, development of, 133, 134
Glomerulonephritis, 141, 142

Glucocorticoids, pharmacological
    effects of, 107, 108
Glycogen storage disorders, 75, 76
Granulomatous disease, chronic, 21, 22
Growth hormones
    binding proteins, 5, 6
    physiology, 3, 4
Growth potential, predictions of, 5, 6
Growth rate and failure to thrive, 155, 156
Guillain-Barré syndrome, 85, 86

Haematology, 59–68
Haematuria, investigation of, 137, 138
Haemodynamic changes at birth, 27, 28
Haemolytic-uraemic syndrome, 15, 16
Haemophagocytic histiocytosis, 67, 68
Haemorrhagic disease of newborn, 63, 64
Hair loss, causes of, 51, 52
Head injury
    child abuse and, 55, 56
    intubation after, 77, 78
Headache, intracranial pathology and, 79, 80
Heart, development of, 129, 130
Heat stroke proteins, 43, 44
Henoch-Schönlein purpura, 93, 94
Hepatoblastoma, 63, 64
Hepatomegaly, 75, 76
Herpes virus type, 6, 11, 12
Hib vaccine, 41, 42
Hirschsprung's disease, 159, 160
Histiocytosis, haemophagocytic, 67, 68
HIV infection
    transmission of, 13, 14
    vaccinations and, 39, 40
Hybridization, 173, 174
Hyper-IgE syndrome, 15, 16
Hyperkalaemia, acute, 69, 70
Hypernatraemia, 137, 138
Hypertension
    causes of, 143, 144
    treatment of pulmonary, 107, 108
Hypocalcaemia, causes of, 75, 76
Hypogammaglobulinaemia, 49, 50
Hypoglycaemia, 165, 166
    causes of neonatal, 73, 74
Hyponatraemia, 71, 72
Hypoparathyroidism, 9, 10
Hypothermia, 73, 74
Hypothyroidism
    congenital, 1, 2
    juvenile, 7, 8
Hypovolaemia and nephrotic syndrome, 145, 146
Hypoxia
    causes of refractory, 31, 32
    ventilator manipulations to improve, 29, 30
Hypoxic-ischaemic encephalopathy, 29, 30

Idiopathic thrombocytopenic purpura, acute, 61, 62
Immunity, syndromes associated with defects of, 49, 50
Immunizations, 39–42
Immunoglobulin, classes and functions, 47, 48
Immunology, 47–50
Incontinentia pigmenti, 53, 54
Incubation periods for infectious diseases, 11, 12
Infections, 11–22
Infectious mononucleosis, 17, 18
Influenza vaccination, 41, 42
Inhalation
    pulmonary complications of, 111, 112
    recurrent, 123, 124
Innervation of upper limb, 83, 84
Insulin, 163, 164
Integumentary system, 135, 136
Intrauterine growth retardation, 23, 24
Intubation following head injury, 77, 78
Intussusception, 161, 162
Iron overload, complications of, 63, 64

Jaundice, cholestatic, 153, 154

Kala-azar, 21, 22
Kawasaki's disease, 13, 14, 21, 22, 61, 62
Ketoacidosis, 165, 166
Kidneys, development of, 135, 136
Klippel-Trenaunay-Weber syndrome, 51, 52

Lamotrigine, 103, 104
Laryngomalacia, 123, 124
Leishmaniasis, visceral, 21, 22

Leukaemia, acute lymphoblastic, 59, 60, 63, 64
Limb hypertrophy, unilateral, 51, 52
Limp, causes of painful, 93, 94
Liver and gastroenterology, 147–62
 nutrition in liver disease, 153, 154
Lungs
 AIDS and, 111, 112
 growth and development, 131, 132
 growth disorders, 125, 126
 therapy for chronic disease, 25, 26
Lupus, features of neonatal, 95, 96
Lymphangiectasis, congenital pulmonary, 121, 122

Macrocephaly, 3, 4
 causes of, 77, 78
Macrocytosis, 61, 62
Malignancies, genes in paediatric, 171, 172
Maple syrup urine disease, 71, 72
Maternal illnesses and neonatal disease, 31, 32
McCune-Albright syndrome, 1, 2
Median nerve, 84
Mediterranean fever, 17, 18
Medium chain acyl coenzyme A dehydrogenase deficiency, 75, 76
Meningitis
 lumbar puncture and meningococcal, 19, 20
 tuberculous, 125, 126
Meningococcal septicaemia, 13, 14
Meningomyelocele, 79, 80
Metabolism, 69–76
 bone disease, 29, 30
 neonatal disorders, 33, 34, 71, 72
Middle aortic syndrome, 177, 178
Miliary tuberculosis, 125, 126
Mitral valve prolapse, 181, 182
Molecular biology, 43–6
Molluscum contagiosum infection, 17, 18
Mumps, 19, 20, 31, 32
'Munchausen by proxy' syndrome, 89, 90
Mycoplasma pneumonia, 123, 124
Myocarditis, 177, 178
 clinical presentation, 179, 180

Nappy rash, 53, 54
Nasal obstruction in infancy, 121, 122

Necrotizing enterocolitis
 clinical features of, 27, 28
 risk factors for development of, 25, 26
Neonatal abstinence syndrome, 27, 28
Neonatology, 23–36
 features of drug administration, 107, 108
Nephroblastoma, 65, 66
Nephrology, 137–146
 see also kidneys; renal
Nephrotic syndrome
 complications of, 143, 144
 hypovolaemia and, 145, 146
Neuroblastoma, 59, 60
Neurology, 77–88
Neutrophil defects and resulting clinical disorders, 47, 48
Nitric oxide, 121, 122
Normal distribution, features of, 101, 102
Nutrition in liver disease, 153, 154

Oesophageal atresia and fistula, 33, 34
Oncology, 59–68
Orthopaedics, 93–100
Osteogenesis imperfecta, 97, 98
Osteomyelitis, bacterial, 95, 96
Osteosarcoma, 99, 100

Pancreatic enzyme insufficiency, 149, 150
Pancreatitis, 153, 154
Parathyroid hormone, 10
Parvovirus B19 infection, 19, 20, 59, 60
Patau syndrome, 171, 172
Patent ductus arteriosus, 181, 182
Pauciarticular juvenile chronic arthritis, 93, 94
Peanut allergy, 47, 48
Periventricular haemorrhage, 25, 26
Periventricular leucomalacia, 33, 34
Peroxisomal disorders, 73, 74
Perthes disease, 93, 94
Pertussis immunization,
 contraindications to, 39, 40
Pharmacokinetics, 105, 106
Pharmacology, 103–10
Phototherapy, complications of, 27, 28
Pituitary gland, development of, 135, 136
Pityriasis rosea, 51, 52
Pityriasis versicolor, 53, 54

Pizotifen, 105, 106
Pneumothorax, 35, 36
Poliomyelitis, vaccination against, 41, 42
Polycystic ovarian disease, 5, 6
Polycythaemia, features of, 29, 30
Polymerase chain reaction, 43, 44
Porphyrias, 151, 152
Pregnancy, drugs contraindicated during, 105, 106
Preterm infant
  apnoea in, 23, 24
  increased risks of, 27, 28
  normal blood count of, 35, 36
Prion diseases, 85, 86
Probability tests, 101, 102
Proteins
  heat shock, 43, 44
  hormone binding, 5, 6
Proteinuria, 141, 142
Prothrombin time, 61, 62
Proto-oncogenes, 45, 46
Prune-belly syndrome, 143, 144
Psoriatic arthritis, 97, 98
Psychosocial paediatrics, 89, 90
Puberty
  delayed, 5, 6
  precocious, 1, 2
  status, 7, 8
Pulmonary hypertension of neonate, drugs for, 107, 108
Pulmonary venous connections, total anomalous, 179, 180
Pupillary signs, pathophysiology and, 79, 80
Purpura, 61, 62
  acute ITP, 61, 62
  Henoch-Schönlein, 93, 94
Pyloric stenosis, 157, 158

Radial nerve, 84
Recurrent inhalation, 123, 124
Reflexes, primitive neonatal, 37, 38
Renal disease, IDDM and end stage, 167, 168
Renal failure, 70
Renal impairment, drugs to be avoided in, 109, 110
Renal physiology, neonatal, 31, 32
Renal stone disease, 139, 140
Renal tubular acidosis, 139, 140
Renal vein thrombosis, causes of neonatal, 143, 144
RNA, 43, 44

Respirology, 111–28
Resuscitation of newborn, causes of failure, 23, 24
Retinopathy, 31, 32
Rett syndrome, 87, 88
Rheumatic fever, 19, 20
Rheumatic heart disease, 175, 176
Rheumatology, 93–100
Rickettsial infections, 17, 18
Rotavirus diarrhoea, 151, 152

Sarcoidosis, 95, 96
Seizures, 81, 82
Severe combined immunodeficiency (SCID), 49, 50
Sexual abuse, signs of, 55, 56
Sexual ambiguity, 7, 8
Sickle cell disease, homozygous, 59, 60
Single gene disorders, 173, 174
Skin rashes, 17, 18
  diffuse erythematous maculopapular, 51, 52
  nappy, 53, 54
  see also purpura
Skull radiology, non-accidental injury and, 55, 56
Spasms, infantile, 81, 82
Statistics, 101–2
Stature
  achondroplasia and, 99, 100
  causes of short, 3, 4
  causes of tall, 1, 2
  height prediction, 5, 6
Steroid therapy
  potential uses of inhaled, 107, 108
  treatment of asthma with, 119, 120
Streptococcus, disorders caused by, 21, 22
Stress, metabolic responses to acute, 75, 76
'Superantigen' disorders, 15, 16
Surfactants
  exogenous, 103, 104
  therapy, 25, 26
Systemic disease, dermatological manifestations of, 53, 54
Systemic lupus erythematosus, 31, 32, 99, 100, 137, 138

Tachycardia, supraventricular, 107, 108, 181, 182

Thalassaemias, 65, 66
  genetic features of, 171, 172
Third cranial nerve palsy, 83, 84
Thrombocytosis, 65, 66
Toxic shock syndrome, 11, 12
Toxicity, drugs and overdose, 105, 106
Tuberculin testing, 41, 42
Tuberculosis
  drugs for, 127, 128
  miliary, 125, 126
Tuberculous meningitis, 125, 126
Tuberous sclerosis, 79, 80
Typhoid, 15, 16

Ulcerative colitis, 159, 160
Ulnar nerve, 84
Urea cycle defects, 73, 74
Urinary tract infection, 143, 144

Vaccination, 39–42
  BCG, 39, 40
  contraindications, 39, 40
  Hib, 41, 42
  influenza, 41, 42
  schedule in England, 41, 42
Varicella infection, complications of, 21, 22
Varicella-zoster immunoglobulin, 41, 42
Ventilation in children, mechanical, 115, 116
Ventilator manipulations, hypoxia and, 29, 30
Visual field defects and neuroanatomical lesions, 81, 82
Vitamin D, 10
Vitamin K, 63, 64
Vomiting, neonatal, 35, 36
Von Willebrand's disease, 67, 68

Wheezing in infancy, 125, 126
Wilms tumour, 66, 139, 140
Wilson's disease, 147, 148

Zellweger's syndrome, 151, 152